Praise for *The California Wine Country Diet*

"People think wine and sumptuous food cannot be a daily part of their lives. But they can, as Dr. Logan teaches"

—John Ash, chef and author of the 2005 James Beard Foundation
Award-winning J*ohn Ash: Cooking One-on-One,*
Private Lessons From a Master Teacher

"...If you love the Wine Country and love reading about it, this is the diet book for you. Plus you get to try out recipes from some of California's edgiest restaurants."

— *San Jose Mercury News*

"Now you can enjoy a "Sideways" wine and food trip through the California wine country while losing weight. What could be better!"

—Nat Ely, executive chef of the Los Olivos Café, featured in the Golden
Globe-winning film *Sideways*

"I can really identify with this book and it's simple and straightforward philosophy. It's as much about taking the time to cook and eat seasonally and locally, and toasting with a good glass of wine, as it is about enjoying everything in moderation. This is a guide for everyone no matter where you live. Cheers!"

—Joanne Weir, chef, author of *Weir Cooking in the Wine Country* and
host of "Weir Cooking in the City"

"The answer to all our dreams...nutritionally balanced, yet pleasurable! Hurrah!"

—Printha Platt, manager, Little River Inn, Mendocino, California

"Balance, diversity, and quality give us the life we hope for, and it is wonderful to find a diet program that embraces this concept."

— Paul Dolan, author of *True to Our Roots,*
president, The Mendocino Wine Company

The California Wine Country Diet *teaches you how moderation doesn't have to be a struggle."*

— Sylvie Greil, Gayot.com

The California Wine Country Diet:

The Indulgent Approach to Managing Your Weight

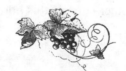

Haven Logan, Ph.D.

Sharon Stewart, R.D.

Quill
Driver
Books

Sanger, California

Published by Quill Driver Books/Word Dancer Press, Inc.
1254 Commerce Blvd.
Sanger, California 93657
559-876-2170 • 1-800-497-4909 • FAX 559-876-2180
QuillDriverBooks.com
Info@QuillDriverBooks.com

Quill Driver Books' titles may be purchased in quantity at special discounts for educational, fund-raising, business, or promotional use. Please contact Special Markets, Quill Driver Books/Word Dancer Press, Inc. at the above address, at Info@QuillDriverBooks.com or at **1-800-497-4909**.

Quill Driver Books/Word Dancer Press, Inc. Project Cadre:
Kathy Chillemi, Mary Ann Gardner, Doris Hall, Stephen Blake Mettee

ISBN: 1-884956-46-7

Printed in the United States of America

QUILL DRIVER BOOKS and COLOPHON are trademarks of
Quill Driver Books/Word Dancer Press, Inc.

To order another copy of this book, please call
1-800-497-4909

Dust jacket photos:
Background photo courtesy Chris Kopack
Inset photo compliments of Fisher Vineyards

Library of Congress Cataloging-in-Publication Data
Logan, Haven.
 The California wine country diet : the indulgent approach to managing your weight / by Haven Logan.
  p. cm.
  Includes bibliographical references and index.
  ISBN 1-884956-48-3
  1. Reducing diets. 2. Physical fitness. 3. Weight loss.
I. Title.
RM222.2.L56 2005
613.2'5--dc22
                                        2005024237

This book is dedicated to those
who have inspired me in this great adventure
about food, wine, and the joys of a healthy life:

My father, Harlan Logan,
who introduced me to the delights of gourmet cooking,

My stepmother, Audrey Logan,
who nurtured me with daily cooking and
never-ending encouragement,

My childhood best friend, Ellen Holmes,
who has shared with me the bliss of food, from
cherry vanilla ice cream on May Apple Road
to the recipes of wine country,

My husband, Robert Faulk,
who first thought up the idea of a diet based on
California wine country cuisine and who has
supported me each step of the way,

My son, Stephen Faulk,
who is far braver in the kitchen than I will ever be,

My patients who have taught me about the complexity
of the emotional and social issues related to food,

And last, but certainly not least, the chefs, vintners,
and food purveyors who dedicate their lives to our
nourishment and pleasure.

Contents

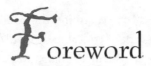

Foreword

by John Ash

What has become known as *California wine country cuisine* has two parts to it. First is a consciousness about where food comes from, with an intention to cook seasonally and locally. The other part is, of course, that it includes wine as a daily beverage! For me, wine is food—it is simply another flavor to enjoy with all the other flavors that are presented on the plate. My role in the evolution of California wine country cuisine was to take on the challenge of educating people—especially Americans, who are a little intimidated by wine—about wine and its role on the table, as well as to help them develop the habit of using ingredients that are locally grown and organic.

California winemakers and chefs initially looked to Europe for inspiration and training. By the late 1970s we had gained enough experience and confidence that we no longer focused on trying to duplicate the wines and foods of Europe. We began to explore our own unique agricultural microclimates and the cuisines of the diverse cultures that had settled in California. In the chefs' recipes in *The California Wine Country Diet* you can see the strong influence of Latin American and Asian, as well as, Mediterranean cuisines.

As a chef, I understand the power restaurants have to influence people and their culinary habits. We have a responsibility not only to present great food but also to make sure we use the best possible ingredients. I belong to an organization called the Chefs Collaborative that has a membership of over one thousand chefs from around the country. We decided a number of years ago that we would get together and promote this idea of a chef's ability to influence how food is grown, produced, processed, and shipped and to support those people who are doing it in the very best way possible. We are encouraging the consumption of what I call "ethical food"—that is, food that is grown by local farmers under organic conditions.

There is truly a revolution going on in the way we look at food. While here in Northern California we are familiar with the idea of consuming locally grown and organic food, this is an idea that is only now catching on elsewhere. As I travel around the country, I find that in large parts of this land the concept of ethical food is still a brand new idea. The proof of this revolution is evident in many ways, such as the setting of national standards for what constitutes a truly "organic" food and the move toward tougher and more comprehensive labeling of food with important information such as the food's country of origin. Ten years ago Americans were not interested in these issues, but more and more they are beginning to recognize that wholesomeness, and not just cost, is important when selecting food. Of course, our continuing concern about health also plays an important role.

The shift away from natural, unprocessed foods began after World War II with the decline of traditional "Leave It to Beaver" households and both parents in a family going to work. "Convenience" became the by-word of the 1950s and 1960s. We were all seduced by it. My parents certainly were. Cooking was seen as drudgery, something you were forced to do, not something you enjoyed doing. That's when the TV dinner was introduced, and fast food restaurants began to spring up everywhere. Today we are still chained to the notion of convenience, and we're not quite sure how to unchain ourselves.

We struggle with contrary notions. On the one hand, we take the attitude in our busy lives that we simply need to fill up our stomachs like we fill up our gas tanks, as quickly and cheaply as possible, which is why we are addicted to fast foods. On the other hand, we have a deep respect for the atmosphere that is created when family or friends gather to eat, drawing together to share a nourishing, home-cooked meal.

My challenge as a chef, and the challenge of people like author Haven Logan, is to educate people about their relationship to food on a personal level, but also on a much larger scale. The foods you choose affect not only your own health but in a very real way also affect the health of the nation, and even the well-being of the globe. Your choices certainly have ramifications for the environment.

When it comes to enjoying food, we have nearly unlimited choices. But we tend to get trapped in trends, such as the recent low-carb trend. People are looking for a "silver bullet" for eating well, maintaining their health, and especially, watching their weight. They think wine and sumptuous food cannot be a daily part of their lives. But they can, as Dr. Logan teaches in this book. We can start eating healthily yet deliciously by choosing a broad range of foods. For instance, farmers' markets have always been an essential part of wine country cuisine. Now there are farmers' markets everywhere, from Wisconsin to Alabama. The cliché that "we are what we eat" is true, and part of a healthy diet and a satisfying culinary experience is to use the freshest ingredients you can and preferably organic ones. Making this one simple change can go a long way toward increasing your well-being and satisfying your palate.

In terms of how to enjoy wine country cuisine while managing your weight, the most obvious solution is to exercise. We should exercise for our health, but we can also be motivated to exercise by rewarding ourselves with excellent food. While it can be a challenge to eat in restaurants and maintain your weight, today there are all kinds of lower-calorie and healthy choices available at most restaurants. If you begin to enjoy cooking, then you can control your calories and also spice up your food choices while cooking at home. Eating well should be part of your life. I have learned that denial is not a long-term solution. At my restaurant, I would hear from diners all the time that the reason they went out to eat was to indulge themselves. Dining out is about pleasure, about pure enjoyment. But that does not mean that you have to sacrifice health or weight concerns in the process. It all comes down to learning to balance your eating habits and your exercise regime.

If there is a single issue in American restaurants today it is portion size. This is of concern to both those running restaurants and to diners trying to combine culinary pleasure with health and weight management. Americans have become used to "value meals," which are huge portions at cheap prices. But what gets sacrificed in the equation is quality, not to mention that we get used to overindulgence and cannot possibly reconcile healthy eating habits and proper weight management. The solution is to eat what you want, but pay attention to portion size.

In my cooking classes, I ask people to guess what the "proper" portion size of the protein on their plate should be. In actuality, it is about the size of your closed fist. But most people guess sizes much larger than that. They say that if they got the proper portion, they would feel cheated, that the restaurant was being stingy with the food. But that is simply a misperception. We generally are not realistic about how much we should be eating. As a matter of course, most people overeat. Europeans, who do not have the obesity problems that we have, eat well while maintaining a more normal body weight. They do not necessarily eat any healthier than we do, but they are much more conscious of the *quality* of their food and the *amount* they consume.

Another aspect of managing weight and maintaining health that has always fascinated me is the pace at which we eat. We claim to want to enjoy delicious food, but we hardly stop to experience the flavor of what we are eating. So, my other advice is to eat more slowly. Your dining experience not only will be much more fulfilling, but you will be helping your body as well. There is a physiological connection between the stomach and the brain. It takes twenty minutes for you to finally begin to have your hunger sated. If you are rushing through your meal, you are not giving your stomach enough time to send your brain the "I'm comfortably full" signal, and you tend to overeat. So, I advise people to prolong the pleasure! Take a little bite of something on your plate and savor it before you take the next forkful. This is a simple behavioral change but a powerful one.

One of the restaurant trends that I think is a healthy one is the movement toward small plates in which there is no so-called main course but a series of small courses. It is a wonderful way to experience not one or two flavors, but a series of many flavors. Sushi, tapas, and dim sum restaurants all fall into this category of dining experience. You can easily reproduce it at home. The satisfaction of so many flavors will increase your sense of satisfaction, and you will not feel deprived even though you will tend to eat less.

It is so much easier today to expand your culinary options than it was even a decade ago. Our supermarkets bring in food from all over the world. Local ethnic markets and farmers' markets abound. There is no reason to be eating "the same old thing" anymore. Cooking cannot be boring when you are experimenting with a world of flavors! If you have not yet taken advantage of the extraordinary range of foods available to you and the easy availability of fresh fruits, vegetables, and fish, then you have a whole new culinary world awaiting you.

Perhaps you are exclaiming, "I'm not a chef!" Not true. Everyone can cook. You only think you cannot cook because you have not really tried. It really is easy. Take green beans. Many people think it is difficult to make "perfect" green beans. But it isn't. Put the green beans in lightly salted boiling water for three minutes, then take them out and drain them. Drizzle them with some good quality olive oil and then season them with a little salt and pepper. To me that is dinner! It is so delicious. You do not even need to use a knife or fork. You can eat them with your fingers!

I am amazed at how savvy many young people are today about food. They have been exposed to the Food Network, celebrity chefs, and the culinary programs in high schools. There is kind of a ground swell of things happening. We have a whole generation of kids coming along who are going to be a lot more confident in the kitchen than previous generations were. Even if you've rarely cooked and never enjoyed it, try your hand at one of the recipes in this book. There are also countless recipes free for the taking on the Internet. Your local library and bookstores are full of cookbooks. Cable television offers many excellent cooking shows. You may be pleasantly surprised to find how much you enjoy both the preparing and the eating of simple, healthy, and delicious meals at home.

Healthy and tasteful food is not processed food. If you make just one change, this would be the one I feel is most important. Stop eating a lot of processed food! When you eat such food you are ingesting all sorts of hidden things that are not especially good for you, such as chemicals and hidden fats. Let's face it—fat is delicious. But the key to enjoying fat is to eat it *consciously.* If you are going to use butter, then allow yourself to taste it! But use it in moderation and in as natural a form as you can.

Unless your health is severely compromised, you can eat basically anything you want if you do it in a balanced and natural way. I call this "mindful eating," and it goes along with eating slowly and enjoying your food. Mindful eating is nothing more than paying attention to what you are eating and how you are eating it. Know what is in your food. Then enjoy every mouthful. In the wine country way of eating, you do not have to deny yourself pleasure to eat in a healthy way.

Described as one of America's most talented chefs and inspirational cooking teachers, and a guiding force in California cuisine, John Ash served for many years as the Culinary Director of Fetzer Vineyards and is on the faculty of The Professional Wine Studies Program at the CIA Greystone. He has a new winery venture called Sauvignon Republic Cellars, specializing in Sauvignon Blanc only. John is the founder of John Ash & Co. restaurant in Santa Rosa and is on the National Board of Overseers of the Chefs Collaborative. He is a recipient of the International Association of Culinary Professionals Cookbook of the Year Award for his book From The Earth to the Table *and the James Beard Foundation Award for* John Ash: Cooking One-on-One.

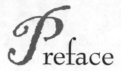# Preface

With *The California Wine Country Diet,* I find myself coming full circle to the excitement I found in food during my childhood. Like many people, as I moved into adulthood, my relationship with food became conflicted. I started to feel that I had to watch everything I ate and give up the foods I most loved if I wanted to be thin and fit. But as a child, I don't remember ever thinking about calories or even knowing anyone who was on a diet. From my perspective today, I can see that some of the foods I ate as a child were not the most nutritious. As John Ash points out in the Foreword, it was the 1950s and we were falling in love with TV dinners. What I do remember was that food was fun. I remember with delight getting to eat all the meringues I wanted by candlelight when a storm cancelled my parents' dinner party. I remember the laughter we shared when my sisters and I competed to see who could prepare the best dinner.

Moreover, my father was a gourmet cook and vice president of General Foods in charge of research and development, so he played a key role in developing all the new convenience foods I, and I am sure many of you, grew to love. Most nights he would bring home an interesting, new food for us to taste test. One night it might be birds' nest soup, and another it might be dehydrated steak that was being tested for use by astronauts. I prided myself on being willing to try any new food.

Leaving home, my food preferences changed. When I moved to the mountains of Mendocino County, California, in the 1970s, I developed a strong interest in what was then known as "health foods." Later, when I moved to Los Angeles to attend graduate school at the University of Southern California, I encountered for the first time the culture of thinness. I decided that I weighed too much and went on my first diet. I lost ten pounds and kept it off during my busy single years. But the struggle with food and diet returned as I approached my late thirties. Even though I kept busy as a wife, mother, homeowner, administrator, and therapist, I found that I was gaining weight and it was harder to take it off and keep it off.

In 1985, I became an administrator at Mt. Diablo Hospital in Concord, California, in charge of the eating disorders and diet and exercise programs. In the next few years I developed a number of other weight-loss programs and provided the psychological support for people following those programs and just about every other program you can imagine, from protein-sparing modified fasts to Weight Watchers to Atkins. All these programs worked in helping people lose weight. The failure came in maintaining that loss over time. As people slowly regained the weight they had worked so hard to lose, they felt discouraged, experienced low self-esteem, and complained of the adverse physical effects of large weight fluctuations.

Spending all my days listening to people worry about their weight, I finally decided just not to think about my own. That solution may have taken some psychological pressure off of me, but it did not help me maintain my weight. Getting older and spending eight hours a day sitting listening to patients, I found the numbers on my scale kept going up.

A few years ago, while in the process of writing my first book, *Choosing to Be Well*, I finally came to accept that if I was going to be in the best health possible, I had to reach and maintain a healthy weight. *The California Wine Country Diet* is the result of that promise to myself and of my twenty years of working with and researching weight issues. I know that this program works, not just because of the research it is based upon and the experience of my patients, but because it has laid the foundation for my own thirty-pound weight loss and maintenance. How glorious it is to wake up each morning feeling vital and twenty years younger in my body!

What's my secret? It is multifaceted, as you will read in this book. But it starts with giving up on the notion that you have to deny yourself the pleasures of food in order to be happy with your weight and body image. Restoring a pleasurable relationship with food is at the heart of the California Wine Country Diet. In addition, especially as we age, we need to be vigilant about our nutrition, the portion sizes of what we eat, and getting enough physical activity. Weight can slowly go up with as little as an extra 100 calories a day. I will show you a variety of ways to make sure you are getting the nutrition your body needs, to monitor your food intake, and to develop a more active lifestyle.

But perhaps the most important aspect of my program is its attention to our emotional relationship with food. Being honest with yourself about your eating patterns and food preferences is essential to changing from eating habits that add to your weight to habits that are conducive to weight loss. Most diets neglect the emotional aspects of eating, and many books on the emotional aspects of eating view them as problems to be overcome. We all need to face the reality that foods and beverages, including wine, are major aspects of our emotional and social lives!

This book will teach you how to enjoy the art of "conscious indulgence." You will learn to combine "conscious" attention to your nutrition, portions, and physical activity with the pleasures of "indulgence" in the foods and life experiences you love. Conscious indulgence is the key to preventing the rebellion and discouragement that usually results from dieting. Conscious indulgence creates the balance that is essential for long-term weight management.

The California Wine Country Diet is an innovative approach to weight management that succeeds because it meets our most basic nutritional and emotional needs in a proactive way. The food of the California Wine Country Diet is not some powder made up in a factory or bland celery and raw carrots. This diet will introduce you to the delicious foods of "California cuisine." You will also be able to eat any other foods you want, albeit in smaller portions. This program will challenge you to examine your reliance on processed foods and to begin to explore the fresh produce available at local farmers' markets, organic groceries, and many supermarkets. By embarking on the California Wine Country Diet, not only will you find it much easier to succeed in reaching your target weight and maintaining it, but you also will be improving your own health and supporting the well-being of our natural environment through your food selections.

at these six aspects of weight management. In Part II, you will begin the implementation of your own diet and physical activity programs while also attending daily to the other four aspects of the wheel. In this section, you will find three weeks of suggested daily food plans for three calorie levels based on the United States Department of Agriculture 2005 Dietary Guidelines for Americans and combined with key points from healthy diets such as the traditional Mediterranean diet and the dishes which have come to be called California cuisine.

At the end of the book you will take a tour through California's various wine growing regions and discover sumptuous recipes from many of the area's finest chefs. Not only will you be able to cook these satisfying and nutritionally sound meals yourself, but also you will better understand the types of restaurant menu items you might want to try when dining out.

While food choices will always be in your hands, I recommend that you try at least two of these new recipes each week. The recipes will add variety and pleasure to your diet, while improving your relationships. (Try it, you'll see what I mean.)

Cooking at home has the benefit of letting you know *exactly* what you are eating. Perhaps also in this process you will discover, or rediscover, the joy of cooking.

Many of the chefs' recipes include food products of the California wine country that are available nationwide. These include certain types of olives, pears, apples, walnuts, sun-dried tomatoes, goat cheese, chocolate, mustard, honey, organic vegetables, fish, and crab. While you might not have tried some of these, one goal of this book is to introduce you to new, pleasurable, and healthy foods, while allowing for your old favorites.

Finally, a unique part of the California Wine Country Diet is the integration of wine into a diet program. The chefs contributing to this book provide suggestions for wine and food pairings with their recipes.

Another aspect of the California Wine Country Diet that is different from most other programs is that it discourages you from obsessing over how quickly or slowly you lose weight. Instead, I ask you to gauge how much more pleasure you are discovering in your life while you are

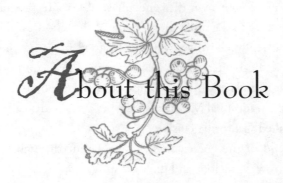

About this Book

Since you picked up this book, I figure you might be wondering exactly what the California Wine Country Diet is all about. In contrast to a typical diet that focuses on how to lose weight as quickly as possible and then leaves you to fend for yourself—which usually means you regain the weight and end up in a vicious cycle of yo-yo dieting—the California Wine Country Diet is a program based on the unique *Wheel of Weight Management*. This wheel includes the six fundamental aspects of healthy weight management:

- Nutrition
- Physical activity
- Practicality
- Pleasure
- Relationships
- Variety.

Rather than focusing only on eating less and exercising more during a "diet phase," with the California Wine Country Diet, all aspects of weight management are emphasized from the beginning and are part of the development of your own individualized program.

This book is divided into two parts. In Part I, you will look in depth losing weight. By taking pleasure in foods that you truly love, moderation is not a struggle. By moving away from denial and giving yourself permission to enjoy food, satisfaction will replace guilty overeating.

The California Wine Country Diet does not promise to be the fastest way to lose weight. What it does promise is to help you with the process of reaching and maintaining a healthy weight in the context of a full and enjoyable life.

PART I

The Wheel of
Weight-Management

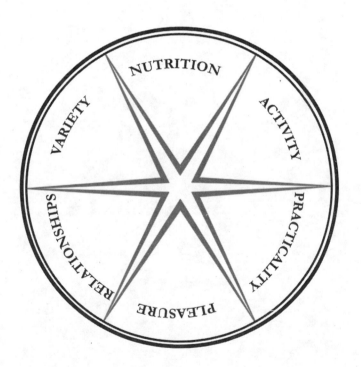

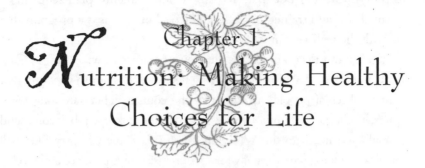

Chapter 1
Nutrition: Making Healthy Choices for Life

" The sensual pleasure of eating beautiful food from the garden brings with it the moral satisfaction of doing the right thing for the planet and for yourself."
—Alice Waters, owner of Chez Panisse

Dinner is served! Your seared wild salmon is accompanied by a fresh green salad with goat cheese, walnuts, and a vinaigrette dressing. On your bread plate is a slice of country bread waiting to be dipped into rich extra-virgin olive oil. Chocolate-covered strawberries will be your dessert. You raise your glass of Pinot Noir with your dinner companion in a toast to another magnificent meal on the California Wine Country Diet!

This scene might be taking place at a restaurant, in the kitchen or dining room of your own home, or out on the deck of a friend's house. Your food choices might be very different from the ones above. While details will differ, this scene illustrates the fundamental principles of the California Wine Country Diet: Taking the time to enjoy freshly prepared, tasteful food in a pleasing environment and in the company of friends and family nurtures us both physically and emotionally. This program demonstrates that a nutritious meal that leads to weight loss does not have to be bland or boring.

The California Wine Country Diet is a unique approach to integrating a wide variety of satisfying and nutritious foods into a healthy physical and emotional life while dropping excess pounds and achieving long-term weight management. It emphasizes a healthy, pleasant, even luxurious culinary lifestyle is not only possible while losing weight and keeping it off, it is essential. Yet this is not a fanciful plan requiring a personal chef and trainer, but a very practical one. This is a program that fits with the reality of modern living.

What tourists do not see as they tour the different wine areas in California is the everyday life of those living here, which is not so very different from the lives of people in the rest of the country. There are long commutes, traffic jams, families to raise, schedules to keep, job layoffs, and generally too much to do. While the California Wine Country Diet will encourage you to take time daily for a leisurely eating experience and weekly for special experiences, it also recognizes that there are times during the week when it may be necessary to eat at the office or even in your car. The challenge of how to eat healthfully on the run is an integral part of the program, and that is why nutrition is the first aspect of the Wheel of Weight-Management that we will look at.

What Should You Be Eating?

Every day we are bombarded with often conflicting and complex information on nutrition and dieting by television, magazines, newspapers, books, and the Web. It is easy to feel confused and overwhelmed, and it is tempting to give up trying to figure out what constitutes a good diet.

In the *California Wine Country Diet* my goal has been to sort through the latest scientific nutritional research for you and place it in the context of delicious California wine country cuisine. No doubt you will come upon studies that contradict some of the recommendations made in this book. Certainly there will continue to be new research published and proclamations from those who claim to have the latest "secret to weight loss." You also may have individual health issues which need to be addressed.

Don't let any of this stand in the way of your achieving a healthier diet. While there is yet to be a consensus on what constitutes the ultimate healthy diet, we are moving in that direction. Keep your eyes on the overall California Wine Country Diet philosophy of eating fresh, local, and seasonal foods while becoming more familiar with the particular recommendations for each food group.

The California Wine Country Diet is based nutritionally in large part on the *Dietary Guidelines for Americans 2005* from the United States Department of Health and Human Services and the United States Department of Agriculture which have been designed to provide "science-based advice to promote health and to reduce the risk for major chronic diseases through diet and physical activity."[1]

Dietary Guidelines for Americans were first published in 1980 and have been revised periodically to stay current with scientific research into health, diet, and nutrition. Due to the rise in obesity over the last twenty years, this latest version of the *Guidelines* contains detailed recommendations about weight management, which are summarized as encouraging "most Americans to eat fewer calories, be more active, and make wiser food choices."[2] The recommendation for those of us who need to lose weight is "to aim for a slow, steady weight loss by decreasing calorie intake while maintaining an adequate nutrient intake and increasing physical activity."[3]

The California Wine Country Diet strongly agrees with this approach. But it will take you beyond purely physical and nutritional concerns, because the single most important factor in your failure or success in losing weight and maintaining your weight loss is not what you eat but the emotional patterns that drive your eating and exercise habits and food and activity choices. While I include many of the government's recommendations—especially about nutrition and exercise—in this book, I will also take you into new territory about what it means to incorporate food and physical activity into a healthier way of living.

Our relationship to food is not intellectual. It is emotional, and it is often driven not by our own thoughts but by opinions that are drilled into us from outside, through advertising and other media and from groups with a special interest in pushing their food products. Even the government is not immune to such pressure. As they designed a new food pyramid in the early 1990s, the USDA and other agencies were lobbied intensely by such organizations as the National Dairy Council, United Fresh Fruit and Vegetable Association, Soft Drink Association, American Meat Institute, National Cattlemen's Beef Association, and the Wheat Foods Council. By allowing such close associations between outside economic interests, the USDA left itself open to the charge that its 1992 food pyramid lacked scientific objectivity. For instance, using that food pyramid as your guide, you would be able to consume up to nine ounces of red meat per day and four and a half cups of ice cream, and to consider french fries as a vegetable. This might be a diet sustainable for a six-foot construction worker who is burning thousands of calories a day in his job, but it is not conducive to good health or weight management for a sedentary office worker.

Given the rapid increase of obesity in this country, it is clear that the 1992, one-size-fits-all food pyramid does not work. The new USDA food pyramid published in April 2005 provides clearer guidelines for different ages, genders, and activity levels. It includes targets for vitamins, minerals, and macronutrients. This new food pyramid can be viewed online at www.mypyramid.gov.

Dietary Guidelines for Americans 2005 stresses consuming a variety of nutrient-dense foods and beverages within and among the basic food groups while choosing foods that limit the intake of saturated and trans fats, cholesterol, added sugars, salt, and alcohol. Daily consumption of four to thirteen servings of fruits and vegetables is recommended compared with a 2000 recommendation of five to nine servings. The 2005 guidelines recommend a daily consumption of three to ten servings of grain products, which should include at least half from whole grains. Consumption of lean meat, fish, and poultry is recommended. Fat consumption is limited to 30 percent of overall calories with less than 10 percent coming from saturated fats. Low trans fat consumption is encouraged. The complete guidelines and a consumer brochure are available online at www.healthierus.gov/dietaryguidelines.

The Cultural Food Pyramids

In addition to the *Dietary Guidelines for Americans 2005*, key nutritional information for the California Wine Country Diet has been gleaned from the various food pyramids developed by Oldways Preservation and Exchange Trust and senior scientists from Harvard School of Public Health, Cornell University, and other institutions. These include the Mediterranean, Latin American, Asian, and vegetarian pyramids. You can find more information about these culture-based dietary programs online at www.oldwayspt.org.

The Mediterranean diet pyramid is the most researched of the cultural pyramids and represents the traditional diet of the island of Crete, much of Greece, and southern Italy as it was known in the early 1960s. The foods that were the basis for a standard diet in this part of the world at that time were non-processed and locally grown. While their diet may have changed over the years, forty years ago people of the Mediterranean tended to eat lots of fruits and vegetables and used meat—particularly lean "white" meat such as chicken and fish—as accompaniments to a meal rather than as the main ingredients. Red meat was eaten only a few times a month. They also ate lots of grains, nuts, seeds, and low-fat cheeses. They got their fat mainly from olive oil. They drank moderate amounts of wine, and physical activity was an integral part of their everyday life.

During their early studies of this diet, the researchers discovered that the people of these areas experienced rates of chronic diseases that were among the lowest in the world and life expectancies that were among the highest, despite the fact that people had limited access to medical care. In September 2004, a study published in the *Journal of the American Medical Association* outlined the health benefits of the Mediterranean diet over the long term. What they discovered was that people who followed this diet and certain lifestyle factors were less likely to develop coronary heart disease, cardiovascular diseases, and cancer. The lifestyle factors contributing to this good health and longevity were nonsmoking, moderate alcohol consumption, and physical activity. The conclusion of the study was that those who followed the Mediterranean diet and the other three lifestyle factors had a 50 percent lower rate of cause-specific mortality.[4]

The Latin American, Asian, and vegetarian food pyramids are each based on the traditional healthy diets of their particular region or eating style. The data showed that people with these kinds of vegetable-rich diets are generally healthier than those of us in more developed countries who eat heavily processed foods and considerably more meat. The California Wine Country Diet takes the best from these recommendations and those of the USDA 2005 Guidelines and places them into a multifaceted approach for both weight management and for finding more pleasure in a healthier lifestyle.

Now let's get back to the basics of this chapter—our nutritional options and choices, which are the foundation of any dietary program.

The California Wine Country Diet
Nutrition Pyramid and Daily Servings

Like the other food pyramids already mentioned, the California Wine Country Diet nutrition pyramid is primarily plant based. It urges you to choose whole grains over refined grains and advises you to incorporate legumes with lean meat or fish sources so that all of your sources of protein are together on one tier. The fat used is primarily from plant sources that are high in monounsaturates, such as olive oil. So it shares a lot with the other pyramid recommendations—until you reach the top of this pyramid. In our pyramid you will find foods and beverages that are not necessary nutritionally but that provide culinary satisfaction and pleasure.

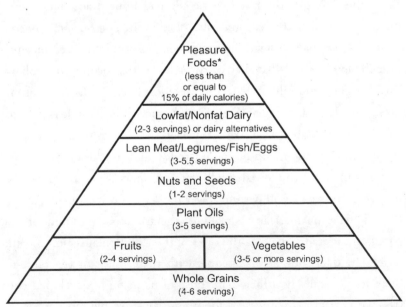

Pleasure Foods*
(less than or equal to 15% of daily calories)

Lowfat/Nonfat Dairy
(2-3 servings) or dairy alternatives

Lean Meat/Legumes/Fish/Eggs
(3-5.5 servings)

Nuts and Seeds
(1-2 servings)

Plant Oils
(3-5 servings)

Fruits
(2-4 servings)

Vegetables
(3-5 or more servings)

Whole Grains
(4-6 servings)

* Pleasure Foods include saturated fats, alcohol, and refined sugar.

*The Nutrition Pyramid and Daily Servings for
1200, 1600, and 2000 Calorie Plans.*

Let's take a close look at certain aspects of nutrition before we examine each tier of the California Wine Country Diet Nutrition Pyramid. The more you know about why certain food choices are being suggested in this program, the more sense it will make for you to shift your habits to include these foods.

Carbohydrates — Tiers 1 and 2 of the Nutrition Pyramid

There are two types of carbohydrates: simple and complex. Simple carbohydrates are called such because they are carbohydrates in their simplest form. They are like the individual bricks of a wall. Simple carbohydrates are also referred to as sugars and are the type of carbohydrate you will find in the fructose in fruit or the lactose in milk. They can also be added to foods at the table or during processing. Complex carbohydrates, on the other hand, are like the brick wall itself. They are a combination of simple carbohydrates combined in intricate ways to form starch, fiber, and glycogen. When completely digested, both simple and complex carbohydrates supply energy to the body—in the form of glucose—to enable your body to move and your brain to think.

It is recommended that 45 percent to 65 percent of our total calories come from carbohydrates, with the majority of these coming from the complex kind. Within this complex type, we also have refined and unrefined complex carbohydrates. The more processed a complex carbohydrate is, the more refined it is. Think of the difference between a wheat berry and white flour. They both start from the same plant, but one is a whole food and the other is refined to a white powder. Unfortunately, in the process of refining carbohydrates we remove the healthy components: fiber, vitamins, and minerals. Unrefined carbohydrates therefore contain more nutrition than their refined counterparts.

The California Wine Country Diet is rich in the complex carbohydrates which are commonly found in what are called "whole foods" such as unrefined grains, fruits, vegetables, nuts, seeds, and legumes. Since whole foods are nutrient dense, they provide a better ratio of nutrients to calories than do refined foods. Whole foods provide the balanced nutrition your body needs, thus potentially minimizing the empty-calorie food cravings you may experience. When your body's needs are met, you feel more satisfied and sated, so you tend to eat less. Eating whole foods not only fills you up faster, it also tends to reduce the amount of calories that are stored as fat. Fat storage depends in large part on how your body processes glucose, or sugar. And when you think of glucose, think of carbohydrates. All carbohydrates when digested break down to glucose, which, as mentioned, provides the fuel for your body to move and your brain to think.

Simple carbohydrates are most often found in processed and convenience foods such as doughnuts, cookies, and the like. They are found in foods that contain refined wheat or bleached flour, such as white bread and pasta. They are also found in foods like white potatoes that are naturally high in glucose. Complex carbohydrates are found in nuts, seeds, legumes, whole grains, fruits, and vegetables.

Simple carbohydrates are processed differently by your body than are complex carbohydrates. When you consume a complex carbohydrate, say a bean burrito, the body has to work to break down the fiber, hull, or skin of the complex carbohydrate—the beans—as its first order of business. This process takes time and so allows for a slow, steady infusion of glucose into your bloodstream. Once your body senses this glucose, your pancreas secretes a synchronized supply of insulin, which signals your cells to absorb the blood glucose for energy or storage. If you are physically active, say walking back to your office from lunch, then the glucose from your bean burrito will go primarily to your leg muscles. If you are mentally active, perhaps studying for an exam, then the glucose will travel primarily to your brain. If, however, you are inactive, let us say you are watching television, then neither your body nor your brain really needs this fuel, so there is no place for the glucose to be used. Instead, your body will store it for later use, when you are active in some way. How does it store it? You guessed it—as body fat.

The problem for most of us, in addition to consuming more "glucose fuel" than our bodies need, is that we tend to consume simple or refined carbohydrates rather than unrefined complex ones. Why is this a problem? Because simple or refined carbs—such as refined breads, cereals, cookies, and regular sodas—take the fast track, instead of the slow track, into our bloodstream. When these types of carbohydrates are consumed, our digestive track does not need to work very hard to process it and move it into our bloodstream because the breakdown work has already been done at the food manufacturer's processing plant. The result is a rapid rush of glucose into the bloodstream. When the pancreas senses this deluge, it overreacts because it does not know how long this floodgate will remain open.

Since the body usually cannot use glucose as quickly as it is being delivered, it will most likely go to—you guessed it again—body fat. In addition, when the pancreas secretes too much insulin, body fat is actually prevented from being converted back into energy. This phenomenon explains why a diet high in refined grains often leads to obesity. In fact, 80 percent of obesity is correlated with a partial mechanical failure of insulin. Moreover, each 5 percent increase in weight during adulthood leads to a 20 percent increased risk of insulin resistance. So, when it comes to carbohydrate consumption, not all carbohydrates are created equal. Unrefined complex carbohydrates are the foods of choice.

Fats — Tiers 3 and 4 of the Nutrition Pyramid

We tend to look at dietary fats as the enemy. But they are not. Fat is essential in the diet because the body needs fats to function properly. It is only when we consume either too much or too little fat that we experience problems such as weight gain or increased risk of certain types of health problems, including coronary artery disease.

We are smart to monitor our fat intake, because fat, by weight, has more than twice as many calories as protein or carbohydrate. This means a certain number of fat calories take up far less "space" than the same number of calories from protein or carbohydrate. For example, 100 calories of butter, a pure fat, fills up less than one tablespoon. But to consume 100 calories of bread, you would have to eat about one to one and a half slices.

Consequently, people who eat high-fat diets tend to exceed their caloric needs and gain weight. Furthermore, people who eat too much fat tend to store body fat more efficiently. Some studies even suggest that people who eat high-fat diets have more body fat than their caloric intakes would predict.

There are two basic types of food fats: saturated and unsaturated.

Saturated fats tend to be solid at room temperature. Examples include butter, coconut oil, beef tallow, palm oil, and lard. Unsaturated fats tend to be liquid at room temperature. Examples include most cooking oils, such as safflower, sunflower, corn, and soybean. A subcategory of unsaturated fats are mono-unsaturated fats, which tend to be liquid at room temperature, but solid when refrigerated. Examples include olive oil, canola oil, peanut oil, and sesame oil.

Other types of fat are hydrogenated fats and trans-fatty acids. Most processed foods contain solid fat in the form of hydrogenated oils. Hydrogenating oil chemically changes a liquid fat to a solid fat. Food manufacturers do this to prolong the shelf life of a product and to improve the texture of foods. For example, a pie crust made with hydrogenated fat is light and flaky, whereas one made with oil can be soggy and dense. The disadvantage of hydrogenated fats is they often contain substantial amounts of trans-fatty acids, which have been shown to increase the risk of heart disease. Major sources of trans-fatty acids include margarine (the hard stick type), snack crackers, cookies, peanut butter (but not the natural kind), and fried foods.

Saturated fats, hydrogenated fats, and trans-fatty acids should be consumed sparingly because consuming too much has been shown to raise LDL-cholesterol, the bad cholesterol. In addition, some epidemiological studies suggest a relationship between specific cancers and these types of fats.

Unsaturated, and primarily monounsaturated fats, are the fats of choice in the California Wine Country Diet because they do not increase risks to your health the way saturated fats do. In addition, they contain the essential omega-3 and omega-6 fatty acids, types of fatty acids needed by the body that can only be supplied by food. A balanced diet that includes grains, seeds, nuts, leafy vegetables, a small amount of vegetable oils, and fish supplies all the omega-3 and omega-6 fatty acids you need.

Protein — Tiers 4, 5, and 6 of the Nutrition Pyramid

Eating adequate amounts of protein is necessary when losing weight, but many weight-loss programs have taken the need for protein to an extreme. Moreover, if you are on a high-protein diet, you are probably also severely restricting your carbohydrate intake. Not surprisingly, this trend in dieting is known as the "high-protein/low-carbohydrate" diet. But here is an interesting point that often gets lost in the hype: Protein has no designated storage sites in the body or brain; so when it is over consumed, it is converted to carbohydrate by the liver. So why do high-protein diets seem to work so quickly? It is mostly because of water loss. Let me explain.

When you begin a high-protein diet, you tend not to eat enough carbohydrates to meet your energy needs, so your body's stored form of carbohydrates—called glycogen—kicks into action to make up for the shortfall. Glycogen needs water in its stored form, and when this energy source is mobilized, so is its accompanying water. And guess what happens then? You lose a large amount of water weight initially.

When the glycogen is used up, your body then looks to its next readily available fuel source—body fat. At first glance you may think, "Great! Melt that fat away!" But there is a dark side. Using fat exclusively for fuel creates by-products called ketones, which in excess create an overly acidic state called ketosis. A classic side effect of ketosis is loss of appetite, which is why the dieter is often able to continue with this type of diet.

However, without the presence of sufficient carbohydrate in the diet, your body will look to its only available source for glucose, your protein stores, to find the glucose it needs to function. In other words, a high protein, low carbohydrate diet does not spare muscle protein from being broken down as often claimed but, in fact, does the opposite.

So there you have it. Any form of severe low-carbohydrate diet provides an initial rapid weight loss of primarily water and lean tissue, and then you are able to continue on the diet because your appetite is suppressed from ketosis. But once you begin to eat a balanced diet again—and not many people can stay on a high-protein/low-carb diet for years—your body will greedily revert to storing glycogen and restoring lean tissue. And you will quickly gain weight—sometimes ending up weighing more than you did when you started your diet.

The California Wine Country Diet program advises that moderation is a better choice than any trendy diet—especially if your goal is lifetime weight management. The simple fact is that eating adequate amounts of protein, but not going overboard with it, is essential for weight loss and long-term weight maintenance.

As with carbohydrates, not all proteins are created equal. There are two types of protein, which are called "complete" or "incomplete." Complete proteins contain all the essential amino acids in relatively the same amounts as your body requires. Generally, complete proteins come from animal foods, like meat, fish, poultry, cheese, eggs, and milk. Incomplete proteins, in contrast, tend to not contain all the essential amino acids and come from plant sources such as beans, seeds, nuts, and grains, such as rice, cereal, and bread.

The good news with proteins is that what one type of incomplete protein lacks, another type has. For example, legumes lack certain amino acids that grains have. In this sense, legumes and grains are complementary proteins. Fortunately, it is not necessary to eat complementary proteins together at the same meal, as long as your protein intake is varied throughout the day and you are meeting your total daily caloric requirements.

Now that we have examined some of the important nutritional aspects of food, let's explore each of the tiers of the California Wine Country Diet nutrition pyramid in detail.

The First Tier of the Nutrition Pyramid: Whole Grains

The California Wine Country Diet recommends 4 to 6 servings per day, depending on your daily caloric intake goal. In Chapter 8 you will figure out which calorie plan you will be on. (One serving = 1 slice bread, 1 ounce dry cereal, or ½ cup cooked hot cereal, pasta, or rice)

At the foundation of our healthy-eating and weight-loss program are whole grains. The emphasis here is on the word *whole*, as discussed in the nutrition section above. On average, Americans consume only one serving of whole grains a day. Their primary grain consumption comes in the form of refined grains. What exactly is a refined grain? Refining refers to the process by which the bran and germ of a grain are removed, leaving only the endosperm. Unfortunately, most of the nutrition also is removed. Don't let the word "enriched" on a package fool you into thinking that a refined grain product is as nutritious as a whole-grain product. Enriching refers to the addition of nutrients to a food to meet a specified standard. Another word for a food that is enriched is "fortified." In the case of enriched or fortified bread or cereal, many nutrients are removed with the bran and germ, yet only four nutrients usually are added back: thiamin, niacin, riboflavin, and iron. Although an enriched or fortified product is better than a non-enriched refined grain product, the truth is that they still lack many other nutrients of a healthy diet, such as vitamins E and B_6, copper, magnesium, zinc, fiber, and a myriad of phytochemicals that are found only in whole grains.

Furthermore, whole-grain products, such as oatmeal and brown rice, not only provide more nutrients and fiber than their refined counterparts, but they also do not contain the sugar that is often added to processed cereals and rice, which adds calories to your daily caloric intake.

The list on page 20 provides a representative sample of some whole-grain and refined-grain food choices. When you have a choice, always opt for the whole-grain product.

Here are some tips to help you get more whole grains each day:

- Stock your pantry with staples made from whole grains: cereal, brown rice, and low-fat whole-wheat crackers, breads, and rolls.
- When eating away from home, select a whole-grain cereal for breakfast.
- Make a habit of requesting foods made from whole grains such as whole-wheat breads and rolls and brown rice as meal accompaniments.
- Check out food labels to help you choose more whole-grain foods each day. Look at both the "Ingredients" list and the "Nutrition facts" panels, and choose foods that list a whole grain as the first ingredient.

The Second Tier of the Nutrition Pyramid: Fruits and Vegetables

*The California Wine Country Diet recommends 2-4
servings of fruit (One serving = 1 medium fruit) and 3 to 5 or*

	Whole grain	**Mostly refined grain**
Grains:	Brown rice	White rice
	Wild rice	
	Buckwheat groats (kasha)	
	Whole barley	Pearl barley
	Quinoa	
	Whole grain bulgur	
	Whole grain pastas	Regular pasta
	Amaranth	
	Ak-mak crackers	Saltines
	Whole wheat bread	White bread, "wheat" bread
	Popcorn (fat free)	Pretzels
Cold cereals:	Cheerios	Basic 4
	Granola or Muesli	Corn flakes
	Grape-Nuts	Frosted flakes
	Nutri-Grain	Just Right
	Raisin Bran	Kix, Corn Pops
	Total	Puffed Wheat
	Wheat Germ	Rice Krispies
	Wheaties	Special K
Hot cereals:	Oat bran	Cream of Rice
	Oatmeal	Cream of Wheat
	Quaker Multigrain	Grits
	Ralston High Fiber	Malt-O-Meal
	Roman Meal	
	Wheatena	

more servings of vegetables per day (One serving = 1 cup raw leafy or ½ cup cooked vegetables).

Fruits and vegetables make up the second tier of your daily food needs, and they an important source of complex carbohydrates. Enough cannot be said about having an abundance of, and a variety of, fruit and vegetables in your diet. Not only are they packed with vitamins, minerals, and fiber, but also they tend to be low in calories. Research has shown that by eating a diet rich in fruits and vegetables, you can decrease your risk for stroke and heart attack, protect against a variety of cancers, lower your blood pressure, better avoid diverticulitis, and guard against cataract and macular degeneration.[5]

The sad truth is that, according to a United States Department of Health and Human Services Centers for Disease Control survey, less than 23 percent of Americans actually eat the recommended minimum "five a day" of fruits and vegetables. In addition, the CDC study reveals that obesity levels are lowest among those people who have high intakes of fruits and vegetables.[6] An added bonus of eating lots of fruits and vegetables is that they provide bulk to your meal thereby inducing a full feeling on fewer calories.

The rule of thumb for getting the most nutrition out of fruits and vegetables is to eat them as close to their natural state as possible. In other words, the more processed they are, the more calories and less nutrition they are likely to have. Compare these two potato products:

	Calories	Fat (gm)	Sodium (mg.)
1 lb baked potato, with skin	440	0.4	32
1 lb potato chips	2,400	162.0	1,230

Another reason to eat fruits and vegetables in their whole form is that they keep us full longer than their processed counterparts. A glass of orange juice leaves the stomach within ten to twenty minutes; an orange with the same number of calories takes significantly longer. The 2005 guidelines recommend eating a variety of fruits and vegetables to provide a wide array of micronutrients and fiber. For example, orange vegetables and fruits like carrots, yams, cantaloupe, and apricots are packed with vitamin A. Dark green leafy vegetables are excellent sources of folate. Citrus fruits are high in vitamin C. By consuming a variety of fruits and vegetables, you will maximize your nutritional intake.

Here are several suggestions for increasing your fruit and vegetable consumption and for improving the choices that you do make:

- Whenever possible make your first choice local, seasonal, and organic. Talk to the farmers at the farmers' market or the produce manager at your supermarket to learn what is in season.
- Expand your palate by trying a new fruit or vegetable each week.
- Grow your own favorite fruits and vegetables.
- Toss cut-up fruit into your green salad for extra flavor, variety, color, and crunch.
- Eat peas out of the pod or small carrots as a snack.
- Cut vegetables ahead of time or buy precut vegetables and salad mixes.
- Add apples, raisins, or pineapple chunks to salads like chicken or tuna.
- Keep a bowl of pre-washed, easy to grab fruit on the counter.
- Take fruit with you every day to work.
- Savor a ripe piece of fruit for dessert.
- Make fruit sorbet. (See the recipe in Chapter 12.)
- When fresh fruits and vegetables are not available, the next best choice is frozen.
- Make a quick smoothie or protein shake using frozen fruit.
- Add frozen mixed vegetables to canned or dried soups.

The Third Tier of the Nutrition Pyramid: Plant Oils

The California Wine Country Diet recommends 3 to 5 servings per day. (One serving = 1 teaspoon of plant oil)

Plant oils are an important part of healthy eating. When researchers studied the Mediterranean diet in the 1960s, they discovered that consumption of olive oil, the principal source of fat in this region of the world, was associated with overall lower levels of chronic diseases and a longer life expectancy. One of the reasons for olive oil's benefits is that it is a monounsaturated fat, which has a neutral effect on serum cholesterol. In other words, olive oil tends to increase HDL-cholesterol levels (the good kind), but has little effect on increasing LDL-cholesterol (the bad kind).

In our culture, olive oil is a healthy choice as a fat in your diet, but it should always *replace* and not be added to other sources of fat, such as butter and margarine. Other monounsaturated-fat oils that can be substituted for unhealthy sources of fats in your diet include canola oil and the oils from avocados, nuts, and seeds.

When making choices about fats, our initial concern is not in terms of calories but in terms of health benefits. All fats have about the same caloric content per serving, about 120 calories per tablespoon. But some fats, as already explained, confer strong health benefits. In terms of dieting, however, the key is to limit your *total* fat intake to no more than 30 percent of your total calories per day. And of that 30 percent, make most of them monounsaturated. The recommendation of 1 to 2 tablespoons of oil a day in the California Wine Country Diet represents the amount that is added to food during cooking or at the table. These amounts are not considered to be a part of your pleasure foods, the last tier, because they are a necessary part of the diet.

The Fourth Tier of the Nutrition Pyramid: Nuts and Seeds

The California Wine Country Diet recommends 1 to 2 servings per day. (One serving = 2 tablespoons of nuts)

Nuts and seeds are excellent sources of protein, fiber, vitamins, and minerals. Nuts in general are very nutritious, providing protein and many essential vitamins, such as vitamin A and vitamin E, minerals such as phosphorous and potassium, and fiber. Although many kinds of nuts contain monounsaturated fats, they still tend to be calorie-rich, so they should be eaten in moderation. Below is a list of the most common nuts and seeds. The ones with an asterisk should be avoided or consumed rarely, as they are high in fat and calories.

Common Nuts	Common Seeds
Almonds	Pumpkin seeds
Brazil nuts*	Sesame seeds
Cashews*	Sunflower seeds
Chestnuts	Flax seeds
Hazelnuts	
Macadamia nuts*	
Peanuts*	
Pine nuts	
Pistachios	
Walnuts	
Filberts	
Soy nuts	
Pecans	
Coconut*	

A rule of thumb when eating nuts or seeds is to measure out no more than two to four tablespoons to eat at one time depending on your calorie plan. Nuts make a great mid-morning or mid-afternoon snack, as they provide the protein and fat to hold you over until the next meal.

Fifth Tier of the Nutrition Pyramid: Lean Meat, Beans (Legumes)

The California Wine Country Diet recommends 3 to 5½ servings per day. (One serving = 1 ounce lean meat or ½ cup of cooked legumes)

This tier makes up the main protein section of the California Wine Country Diet nutrition pyramid. This category includes poultry, eggs, fish, legumes, lean pork, and lean red meat. Unfortunately, many protein-rich foods are often fat-rich foods that contribute to obesity. For this reason, the foods recommended in this tier of the California Wine Country Diet nutrition pyramid have adequate levels of protein without the added fat. It is important to consume a variety of these proteins throughout the week to obtain a broader range of nutrients rather than focusing on just one or two.

Legumes are another name for beans and peas, such as lentils and kidney, pinto, navy, and lima beans. These foods are excellent sources of plant protein and also provide other nutrients such as iron and zinc, although the iron in legumes is not as readily absorbed as the iron in lean red meat. In addition, they are excellent sources of dietary fiber and nutrients such as folate that are low in the diets of many people. One-half cup of cooked legumes is considered one serving.

Fish is not only an excellent source of protein, but many types of fish are also rich in omega-3 fatty acids, which may help reduce the risk of heart disease. Preparing fish by broiling or poaching keeps the added fat to a minimum. Poultry, such as chicken, turkey, and Cornish game hens, is also a relatively low-saturated fat source of protein, if you do not eat the skin.

One of the most complete and digestible proteins is egg protein. Eggs also contain a highly absorbable form of lutein, a nutrient thought to protect against cataracts and age-related macular degeneration. Eggs have been demonized for contributing to high blood-cholesterol levels. Granted, they contain a substantial amount of dietary cholesterol, but remember, it is the saturated fat that increases our blood cholesterol, not dietary cholesterol. The average egg contains one-third the saturated fat of an ounce of cheese. So, in fact, eating an egg has less of an effect on blood cholesterol than eating a piece of cheese. One egg is considered one protein serving.

For many people, especially those who have been on a high-protein/low-carbohydrate diet, adjusting to the lower amount of protein recommended by the 2005 *Guidelines* and the California Wine Country Diet may be difficult. As you learn to make protein an "accompaniment" on your plate rather than the center of it, two strategies can help you in the transition. One is to use some of your pleasure food calories for additional ounces of eggs, meat, fish, or beans. The other is described below—shifting a dairy serving to a lean meat serving if you have provided for your calcium needs that day with calcium supplements.

The Sixth Tier of the Nutrition Pyramid: Low-Fat and Non-Fat Dairy Products or Calcium Supplements

The California Wine Country Diet recommends 2 to 3 low or nonfat dairy servings per day or with no dairy add three 500mg of calcium supplements per day. Each dairy serving you do not consume can be exchanged for an ounce of protein on tier 5.

When we think strong bones and teeth, we think calcium from dairy products. However, many people do not drink milk, whether because of lactose intolerance or because they just do not like it. But there are other ways to get calcium than from milk, one cup of which in its whole form contains as much saturated fat as four strips of bacon. (Milk alternatives are described later in this section.) If you enjoy dairy products, stick to low-fat or nonfat choices, such as nonfat or 1-percent milk, nonfat yogurt, and low-fat or nonfat cheese (the low-fat varieties generally have less than five grams of fat per ounce).

Alternative ways of obtaining adequate calcium include nondairy sources of calcium such as calcium-enriched juice, lactose-reduced milk products, dark green leafy vegetables, canned fish with bones, and tofu with calcium sulfate. You can take lactase enzyme (Lactaid) before consuming milk products or switch to lactose reduced milk products to minimize any lactose-intolerance problems.

If you do not consume dairy products at all, then calcium supplements are an easy way to get your daily calcium requirement. Aim for 1,200 to 1,500 mg of *total* calcium a day. The best form of calcium supplement in terms of absorption is calcium citrate malate, followed by calcium carbonate. If supplementing, have one supplement in the morning and one later in the day or evening to maximize absorption, preferably with food.

Top of the Nutrition Pyramid: Pleasure Foods

Recommendations for the first six tiers of the nutrition pyramid have been listed in number of servings. At the top of the Pyramid we will switch to calories in order to give you the freedom to make selections from any food group you wish. The California Wine Country Diet recommends that no more than 15 percent of your daily calories come from the pleasure foods category. In Chapter 8 you will figure out which calorie plan you will be on and how many pleasure food calories you can have each day.

An important feature in the California Wine Country Diet nutrition pyramid is the incorporation of what I call "pleasure foods," which will be different for each of us. Most weight-loss regimens eliminate foods that contain ingredients key to these pleasure foods, namely, saturated fat, refined sugar, and alcohol. It is the California Wine Country Diet philosophy that foods or beverages that contain these ingredients need not be avoided completely, but rather can be consumed in amounts that will still allow you to reach your weight-loss and weight-management goals.

I advocate *conscious indulgence,* which is a responsible way of allowing yourself your preferred foods in moderation. You can allow yourself your favorite culinary pleasures, but in amounts that will not affect your health or weight management goals in a negative way. If you are a chocolate cake lover, you can have an occasional piece, but you cannot eat the whole cake in one sitting!

The California Wine Country Diet nutrition pyramid is designed to help you discover a healthier way of eating for a lifetime, not just for short-term weight loss. This program allows you to avoid relapse and yo-yo dieting, because it allows you eat the foods you love but that are typically forbidden in other weight-loss programs.

The government's *Guidelines 2005* has introduced a similar concept in what is called very generally "discretionary calories." In the California Wine Country Diet nutrition pyramid, however, there are three specific types of pleasure foods at the top of the pyramid: foods with saturated fat, alcohol, and sugar. You should plan for 15 percent or less of your total calories per day coming from this tier. For example, if you need to consume 1,600 calories a day to lose weight, then 240 calories or less (1,600 x 15 percent) should come from the pleasure foods category.

What are some common examples of about 200 calories of a pleasure food? About 1½ tablespoons butter, four ounces of lean red meat, two light beers, ten ounces of wine*, two homemade chocolate chip cookies, or one and a half ounces of semisweet chocolate.

The inclusion of pleasure foods in this program helps you to say good-bye to will power and hello to conscious indulgence. Most people who easily manage their weight already practice this behavior naturally. They enjoy their treats, savoring each bite, but then they move on to other foods that provide their basic nutrition.

Only you can make the choices that will make your diet successful. While you can learn from the experiences and expertise of others, what works for you will be unique to you. The key is in realizing that permanent weight management requires permanent ways of thinking and behaving. The changes you make need to be ones you can live with for the rest of your life.

Losing weight and keeping it off means stopping or modifying those behaviors that contribute to weight mismanagement and doing the things that contribute to weight management. The California Wine Country Diet is a program that spends more time on these other factors than it does on food precisely because it is in these others areas that we most often meet failure or discover success when trying to lose weight or maintain our weight.

Nutrition is the first of the six aspects of the Wheel of Weight-Management. In the following chapters of Part I, we will examine the

---

A word about alcohol—If you choose alcohol as your pleasure food, then be aware that health care researchers recommend that alcohol should be limited to no more than one drink per day for women and two drinks per day for men. When consumed in these amounts, alcohol may have beneficial health effects, but beyond these amounts harmful effects can result. Of course, a woman should never drink alcohol if she is pregnant, plans to become pregnant, or is lactating. Nor should anyone consume alcohol if he or she is taking medications that could interact with it, have specific medical conditions that can be exacerbated by the consumption of alcohol, or if that person feels he or she will have trouble restricting alcohol intake. Never consume alcohol when operating machinery or driving a car.

other five areas that will contribute to your success: activity, practicality, pleasure, relationships, and variety. Each of the six aspects contributes in its own unique way to a richer life in which managing your weight will no longer be an ordeal.

Chapter 2
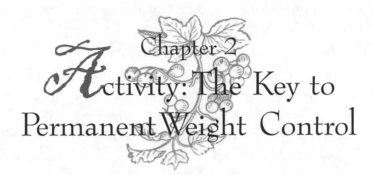Activity: The Key to Permanent Weight Control

"Overweight persons are better characterized as under exercised rather than overfed."
　　　　　—Steve Blair, Ed.D., Director of Research,
　　　　　Cooper Institute, Dallas Texas

Extremely discouraged after numerous weight-loss attempts, a new client I will call "Joan" told me, "I've tried every diet out there over the last twenty years and nothing has worked." She filled me in on her struggle with weight. When she was first married, she weighed 135 pounds. After the birth of her second child, her weight ballooned to 180 pounds, which is when she decided to make a concerted effort at weight loss. Over the years, she made at least fifteen weight-loss attempts, trying just about every type of diet program and even weight-loss medications. Each time she was successful, she lost an average of twenty-five to thirty pounds. But then the weight would creep back on; she would regain an average of thirty to thirty-five pounds. When she finally came to see me, she weighed 290 pounds, 155 pounds more than when she was first married.

As I talked with Joan I asked the question that makes most of my clients—and just about everyone who is hoping to lose weight—cringe: "How much exercise did you incorporate into your weight loss program?" Joan replied sheepishly but honestly, "As little as I could get away with."

Joan's story is a classic case of yo-yo dieting, or the continual losing and regaining of weight. While most dieters experience this vicious and frustrating cycle, they do not understand why it happens. So, let us begin this chapter by examining the yo-yo syndrome.

Yo-Yo Dieting and Physical Activity

The reason Joan gained a little more weight each time is because of what happens to body composition and metabolic rate during and after weight loss. Physical activity is at the heart of this process. Before Joan lost her first twenty-five to thirty pounds, she was maintaining her weight by eating about 2,500 calories per day. During her first diet, she limited her calories to 1,500 a day, for a 1,000-calorie deficit from her normal eating habits. She lost about two pounds a week and was feeling great. However, since Joan did not incorporate much exercise, her weight loss was not entirely fat. Some of the loss was from loss of lean tissue, or muscle. By losing lean tissue, Joan was reducing her metabolic rate.

The more muscle you have, the higher your metabolic rate and the more easily you are able to burn calories, even when doing nothing. In fact, every pound of muscle burns about thirty-five calories per day.[1] One pound of fat, on the other hand, burns only three calories per day. Imagine two friends: Joe weighs 200 pounds and has 15 percent body fat. Frank also weighs 200 pounds, but has 30 percent body fat. When sitting down together to watch a football game, Joe will burn more calories than Frank just because he has more lean tissue. Preserving lean tissue is even more important during weight loss than at other times, because it is the key to keeping your engine revved, so to speak, which allows your body to burn additional calories, even while you are at rest.

Studies have shown over and over again that when you lose weight by diet alone, more lean body mass is lost than when weight is lost by diet combined with exercise. *The fact is you can only maintain or build lean tissue with exercise.*

This brings us back to Joan. When she had reached her weight goal, she slowly reverted to her 2,500-calories-a-day eating pattern. Of course, she began to regain the weight she had lost—and then some, because 2,500 calories was more than her newly slimmed body needed. But when she started to diet again, she found that to lose weight she had to cut back her calorie intake even further, to about 1,200 calories a day, because she had failed to build up her lean tissue. You can see how, if this pattern continues over the years, it leads to a common complaint from frustrated dieters: "I hardly eat anything, yet I can't lose weight!"

If you find yourself in a similar situation to Joan's, all is not lost. Yes, you are starting at a metabolic disadvantage, in that your body has become a very inefficient user of calories. However, with the incorporation of the right amount of exercise, you can increase your metabolic rate and therefore your fat-burning potential.

Exercise for Permanent Weight Control

Almost 70 percent of American adults do not exercise regularly, and of these, 35 percent to 40 percent do not exercise at all.[2] Yet, exercise is so important for weight loss and weight maintenance that it has been identified as one of the key behaviors among people who have kept the weight off.[3] Results of a three-year study demonstrated that individuals who exercised as part of their weight-loss program showed better long-term weight loss compared with those who only dieted. During the follow-up period, those who exercised continued to lose or maintain their weight loss, but those who only dieted began to steadily regain the weight.[4]

There is no getting around the facts: Exercising as part of a weight-loss program pays off in big ways. In any reducing plan, with or without exercise, in the first three days, approximately 70 percent of the weight loss will be water, only 25 percent fat, and the remainder lean tissue. However, when exercise is incorporated, by about the second week, 69 percent of weight loss is fat. By the third week, 85 percent of the weight loss is fat. Who wouldn't love those results? But now consider the results if you diet without exercising: Only 55 percent to 65 percent of your weight loss will be fat.[5] The payoff of exercise is that you are training your body to use fat as fuel.

What's more, exercise also makes you feel good. When you feel good about yourself, you are less likely to want to continue behaviors that do not promote good health. In fact, the main reason that active people exercise is because it makes them feel good—and not just during their exercise, but after. This can happen to you also. One of the key benefits of feeling better while losing weight is that it motivates you to eat better.

Desires to overeat or binge fade away; you are more apt to choose an apple over chips as a snack, for example. Think of exercise as the internal support you need to eat better, feel better, and look better.

If these reasons are not enough to get you thinking about the benefits of exercise, here are a few more:

- Improved quality of sleep
- Sharper mental alertness
- Less depression
- Improved self-esteem
- Improved self-discipline
- Shapelier figure
- Improved appearance
- Increased mobility, flexibility, reaction time
- Improved immunity to disease
- Decreased risk of chronic diseases (diabetes, heart disease, cancer)
- Prevention or reduction of bone loss in postmenopausal women
- Decreased smoking and alcohol use
- Improved sexual performance
- Slowing of the aging process

The bottom line is this: *To lose weight and keep it off, you have to make exercise an integral part of your life.* If you are thinking you can get away with very little physical activity, you are only fooling yourself. Like any habit though, with consistency and a positive attitude you can change your old patterns or replace them with new ones. You *can* become a more active person, and in all likelihood, you will even find you enjoy the new you!

Assessing Your Level of Physical Activity

Here's a questionnaire developed by the Canadian Society for Exercise Physiology that will help you decide if you should consult with your health-care professional before embarking on an exercise regime.

Physical Activity Readiness Questionnaire — PAR-Q*6
PAR-Q & You

(A questionnaire for people aged 15 to 69)

Regular physical activity is fun and healthy, and increasingly more people are starting to become more active every day. Being more active is very safe for most people. However, some people should check with their doctor before they become much more physically active.

If you are planning to become much more physically active than you are now, start by answering the seven questions below. If you are between the ages of 15 and 69, the PAR-Q will tell you if you should check with your doctor before you start. If you are over 69 years of age, and you are not used to being very active, check with your doctor. Common sense is your best guide when you answer these questions.

Please read the questions carefully and answer each one honestly.

Yes	No	
❏	❏	1. Has your doctor ever said that you have a heart condition *and* that you should only do physical activity recommended by a doctor?
❏	❏	2. Do you feel pain in your chest when you do physical activity?
❏	❏	3. In the past month, have you had chest pain when you were not doing physical activity?
❏	❏	4. Do you lose your balance because of dizziness or do you ever lose consciousness?
❏	❏	5. Do you have a bone or joint problem (for example, back, knee, or hip) that could be made worse by a change in your physical activity?
❏	❏	6. Is your doctor currently prescribing drugs (for example, water pills) for your blood pressure or heart condition?
❏	❏	7. Do you know of any other reason you should not do physical activity?

---

* Informed use of the PAR-Q: The Canadian Society for Exercise Physiology, Health Canada, and their agents assume no liability for persons who undertake physical activity, and if in doubt after completing the questionnaire, consult your doctor prior to physical activity.

Yes to One or More Questions

If you answered *yes* to one or more questions, talk with your doctor by phone or in person before you start becoming more physically active or before you have a fitness appraisal. Tell your doctor about the PAR-Q and the questions where you answered *yes*.

- You may be able to do any activity you want—as long as you start slowly and build up gradually. Or, you may need to restrict your activities to those which are safe for you. Talk with your doctor about the kinds of activities you wish to participate in and follow his or her advice.
- Find out if supervised community exercise programs are available and which might be safe and helpful to you.

No to all questions

If you honestly answered *no* to *all* PAR-Q questions, you can be reasonably sure that you can:

- Start becoming more physically active—begin slowly and build up gradually. This is the safest and easiest way to go.
- Take part in a fitness appraisal—this is an excellent way to determine your basic fitness so that you can plan the best way for you to live actively. It is also highly recommended that you have your blood pressure evaluated. If your reading is higher than 144 over 94, talk with your doctor before you start becoming much more physically active.

Delay Becoming Much More Active:

- If you are not feeling well because of a temporary illness such as a cold or fever, wait until you feel better.
- If you are or may be pregnant, talk to your doctor before you start becoming more active.

If your health changes so that you then answer *yes* to any of the above questions, tell your fitness or health professional. Ask whether you should change your physical activity plan.

International Physical Activity Questionnaire[7]

This questionnaire was developed to assess your level of physical activity. Answer the questions in terms of your physical activities in the last seven days. Include activities you do at work, as part of your house and yard work, to get from place to place, and in your spare time.

1. During the last seven days, on how many days did you do vigorous physical activities like heavy lifting, digging, aerobics, or fast bicycling?

    _____ days per week
    _____ no vigorous physical activities; skip to question 3

2. How much time did you spend doing vigorous physical activities on one of those days?

    _____ hours per day
    _____ minutes per day

    Think about all of the moderate activities that you did in the last seven days. Moderate activities refer to activities that take some but not a lot of physical effort and make you breathe somewhat harder than normal. Think only about those physical activities that you did for at least ten minutes at a time.

3. During the last seven days, on how many days did you do moderate physical activities like carrying light loads, bicycling at a regular pace, or doubles tennis? Do not include walking.

    _____ days per week
    _____ no moderate physical activities; skip to question 5

4. How much time did you spend doing moderate physical activities on one of those days?

    _____ hours per day
    _____ minutes per day
    _____ don't know/not sure

Think about the time you spent walking in the last seven days, including at work and at home, getting from place to place, and any other walking that you might do solely for recreation, sport, exercise, or leisure.

5. During the last seven days, on how many days did you walk for at least ten minutes at a time?

    _____ days per week
    _____ no walking; skip to question 7

6. How much time did you spend walking on one of those days?

    _____ hours per day
    _____ minutes per day
    _____ don't know/not sure

Scoring:

Multiply the total number of minutes and the total days per week for each type of activity by the following numbers to get your point scores for each activity:

	Total Days		Total Minutes			Points
Vigorous:	_____	x	_____	x	8.0 =	_____
Moderate:	_____	x	_____	x	4.0 =	_____
Walking:	_____	x	_____	x	3.3 =	_____
					Total	_____

Very Active

If your number of Vigorous activity points is at least 1,500, *or* you did seven days of a combination of all three levels of physical activity for a minimum of 3,000 points, you are already physically active and should have no problem reaching your weight goal. The key issue for you will be monitoring your food intake to create a calorie deficit.

Minimally Active

If you did vigorous activity three or more days a week for at least 20 minutes per day *or* walking or moderate activity five or more days a week for at least 30 minutes per day *or* any combination of walking, moderate, or vigorous activity five or more days a week for a minimum of at least 600 points, you are minimally active. You have a good baseline but need to develop an even more active lifestyle to permanently manage your weight.

Inactive

If you reported no activity *or* less that 600 points, you need to get moving. You will not lose weight and keep it off unless you do so. By starting with what you can do, and gradually building on your progress, you can and will develop an active lifestyle.

How to Develop a More Active Lifestyle

"It's OK not to be an athlete. It's not OK to be a couch potato."
— *Laura Pawlak, Ph.D., M.S., R.D.*

Change is not easy, especially if it involves doing something that does not sound like a whole lot of fun. However, you do not have to become an Olympic athlete to fit the mold of an exerciser. You just need to be able to do the necessary amount to allow your body to lose weight at a healthy rate. When it comes to exercise, the following steps will help you to become a lifetime exerciser:

1. *Identify activities you enjoy doing and think you can do with relative ease.*

What you enjoy doing is unique to you. When deciding what you may enjoy, think of the types of activities that appeal to you and what you feel confident in being able to do.

- Do you like to be alone? Then choose solo exercises such as walking, jogging, hiking, biking, swimming, aerobics at home, and exercise machines.
- Do you like the camaraderie of a group? Consider taking an aerobics class, training for a running race, Masters Swimming, joining

a walking or running club or an organized group training for an event (e.g., Team in Training).

- Do you prefer the companionship of just one? Find a walking buddy (even your dog!), spot a friend when weight training, or find a friend to take an aerobics class with you.
- Are you competitive? Think basketball, volleyball, tennis, or racquetball. Train for a marathon or triathlon.
- Do you like quiet, low-impact activity? Try yoga, Pilates, or Tai Chi.

If you are able to identify activities that appeal to you, the more likely it is that you will be able to stick with them.

2. *Identify potential barriers to exercise and overcome them.*

Barriers to exercise come in many forms. Identifying your barriers is the first step in overcoming them. Below are some of the most common barriers to exercise. Circle the ones that might come up for you:

Poor attitude towards exercise	Physician's advice
Lack of control over your life	Access to exercise
Lack of self-confidence with exercise	Bad weather
Lack of time	Inertia
Discomfort associated with exercise	Isolation
Physical limitations	Fear of injury

Overcoming your obstacles may take time and effort on your part. Just because you have identified some barriers, do not give up on the idea that you can grow to love, or at least like, exercising. Below are some effective solutions for barriers:

- Think positive. Remember the positive benefits of exercise (fun, excitement, companionship, stress control, feeling better, looking better, improved health).
- Keep it simple. Choose activities that require little organization, equipment, financial expenditure, or contact with, or cooperation from, other people.

- Find ways to overcome barriers to exercising: Buy in-home equipment, exercise videos, or rain gear. Make a commitment to a walking buddy who will expect you to show up, and so on.
- Maximize convenience: Lay out your exercise clothes the night before, alter your route home so you go by the gym, place a treadmill in your office.
- Enlist help or support if necessary. There may be solutions to your barriers that you may not have thought of. Perhaps you will need to find motivation by hiring a personal trainer to teach you proper exercise techniques or see a counselor to help you in reassessing your life's priorities. Most aversion to exercise is mental, not physical.

3. *Program exercise into your life.*

Like brushing your teeth, exercise must become a regular part of your life. For some of you who do not exercise regularly, this may mean programming your life in a way you have never done before. It takes about half a year to "lock in" a new behavior, so be prepared to dedicate yourself to becoming more active for a minimum of six months. If you do that, you are much more likely to make exercise a part of your life, permanently.

Get out your calendar and write in the days and times you will exercise, in ink. Keep these appointments with yourself and let nothing interfere. If you skip a few days due to illness, work schedule, or other obligations, the sooner you get back into the exercise groove, the more likely you will be able to get back into your routine. If you continue to skip days, the more likely it will be that you will abandon your program altogether. By scheduling your exercise, you cannot miss a workout because it is already structured into your week. If you take a more lax attitude, other things easily will take the place of your exercise plans.

4. *Monitor your progress.*

Monitoring your progress is a strong motivator to keep you on the active path. When you can see where you started and then evaluate how far you have come, you have a powerful tool that provides feedback on your progress, helps prevent boredom, and keeps you accountable. One way to monitor your progress is by keeping an activity log. Use the log to keep track of your achievements, such as minutes walked, pounds lifted, and heart rate. Another useful tool is a heart-rate monitor. As you will learn in Chapter 7, "Starting Your Activity Program," your heart rate is your most effective tool for monitoring your change in fitness. You will find that with time, you will be able to exert more effort at a lower heart rate.

5. *Reward yourself for small goals reached along the way.*

We all like to treat ourselves now and then, but when you tie rewards into goal-achieving behaviors, that behavior is more likely to be reinforced. In the short term, you can make your own rules, that you cannot do some other activity for example, until you do your exercise. For example, you cannot take a shower until you take your morning walk. In the long run, you may want to reward yourself with some treat such as a massage or facial for reaching milestones in your fitness goals. You deserve it!

The Activity Pyramid

Similar to the California Wine Country Diet nutrition pyramid, the activity pyramid is made up of tiers that represent the seven components of an active lifestyle: activities of daily living, aerobic activity, flexibility, balance, strength training, anaerobic activity, and rest. Before we get to the individual tiers of the pyramid, however, let's take a look at how much exercise is enough exercise.

How Much Is Enough?

The *Dietary Guidelines 2005* state that in order to lose weight, you will need to "participate in at least 60 to 90 minutes of daily moderate-intensity physical activity while not exceeding caloric intake requirements."[8]

This is much more time than previously thought; yet data from the National Weight Control Registry shows that individuals who maintained weight loss for an average of five years exercised at least an hour a day. This finding was echoed in a concurring recommendation by the Institute of Medicine, a part of the National Academy of Sciences that advises the government. In addition, the 2005 *Guidelines* state that to prevent unhealthy weight gain, you need to get approximately 60 minutes of moderate-intensity to vigorous-intensity physical activity on most days of the week. At first glance, this recommendation may seem impossible for you to follow. However, a closer look at the definition of moderate-intensity exercise puts this recommendation in a more realistic light.

According to the U.S. Department of Health and Human Services Centers for Disease Control and Prevention and the American College of Sports Medicine, this recommendation includes any activity that burns 3.5 to 7 calories per minute.[9] Granted, what constitutes moderate intensity is completely subjective depending on many factors including your level of fitness and age. For example, what is *moderate* to a fit twenty-year-old might be *vigorous* to a sixty-year-old sedentary person. Generally, activities like those mentioned below that you can do for at least 25 minutes without tiring would be considered moderate:

- Moderate or brisk walking, 3 to 4.5 mph
- Cycling, 5 to 9 mph
- Dancing: aerobic, ballroom, folk, modern

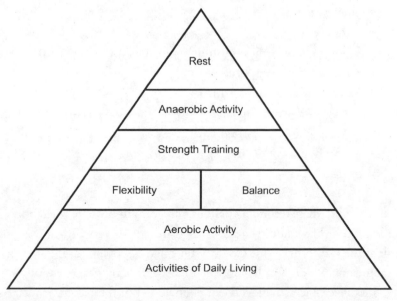

The Activity Pyramid

- Yoga
- Weight training
- Light calisthenics
- Doubles tennis
- Swimming, recreational
- Gardening and yard work (raking, hoeing, weeding, pushing a power lawn mower)
- Moderate housework (scrubbing floors, sweeping, washing windows)

Depending on your fitness level, you may also include in this 60 to 90 minutes any *vigorous* activity, which typically are activities that you could keep up for less than 25 minutes, such as:

- Racewalking, 5-plus mph
- Jogging or running
- Backpacking
- Bicycling, 10-plus mph
- Dancing: high impact, step aerobics; energetic ballroom, folk, or square dancing
- Singles tennis
- Jumping rope
- Vigorous calisthenics (push-ups, pull-ups, jumping jacks)
- Most competitive sports
- Swimming steadily paced laps
- Heavy yard work (digging, swinging an ax, hand-splitting logs, pushing a non-motorized lawn mower)
- Heavy housework (carrying 25 lbs or more upstairs, moving furniture)

As I said, these recommendations may seem impossible when printed before you in black and white. But they are not so very difficult. If you look at the California Wine Country Diet activity pyramid, the tiers that contain activities of daily living (ADLs), aerobic activities, strength training, and anaerobic activities all can be included in the recommended 60 to 90 minutes. For example, if you walked for 30 minutes, did 30 minutes of ADLs throughout the day, and strength trained for 15 minutes, you would easily meet the 2005 *Guidelines* for physical activity and fulfill the first four tiers of the California Wine Country Diet activity pyramid. Let us now look at the pyramid in more detail.

First Tier of the Activity Pyramid:
Activities of Daily Living

Activities of Daily Living make up the foundation of the activity pyramid. These are activities you do as part of your regular day, like walking to and from your car, lifting groceries, climbing a flight of stairs. Unfortunately, technological conveniences have reduced the number or frequency of ADLs we perform each day. For example, cars, buses, subways, elevators, escalators, and moving sidewalks in airports reduce the number of steps we take each day. Remote controls, drive-thru restaurants, even electric can openers reduce our need to move or exert physical effort. If you compare your activity level today with that of a man or woman of only fifty or 100 years ago, you will quickly see how many fewer calories you need as fuel to live your life. Couple that reality with the fact that we tend to eat many more calories than our ancestors did and you can see why the majority of us have weight problems.

We certainly do not want to give up our modern conveniences, but we do need to be realistic about the effects of our decreased energy expenditures on our weight and our fitness levels. By incorporating more movement into your activities of daily living, you begin to increase the number of calories you burn and increase your capacity to lose weight. So, you need to become conscious of how you can do that—not only on a daily or hourly basis, but on a minute-by-minute basis as well.

Here are a few ideas. Add your own to this list.

- Park at the back of the lot at the supermarket.
- Load your own groceries into the car.
- Get up and change the channels on your television.
- Take an activity break instead of a snack break at the office.
- Walk around the room when talking on the phone rather than sitting.

- Play with your kids.
- Take the stairs instead of the elevator or escalator. If you are going up many floors, take the first few flights of stairs, and then take the elevator.
- Mow the lawn with a push mower rather than a riding tractor mower.
- Walk or ride a bike instead of driving short distances.
- Get off the bus or subway one stop early and walk the rest of the way.

Your goal is to work up to at least three hours a week, or about 30 minutes a day, of increased ADLs.

Second Tier of the Activity Pyramid: Aerobic Activity

Aerobic activity is the kind of movement that gets your heart pumping a little more than ADLs, but not so much that you feel out of breath. It is also the kind of activity that tends to be done on a consistent basis, as part of a routine. Examples of aerobic activity include:

- Brisk walking
- Jogging or running
- Cross-country skiing
- Bicycling
- Dancing
- Vigorous ball sports (volleyball, basketball, racquetball, singles tennis, squash, handball)
- Stair climbing
- Skating
- Swimming
- Aerobic dance

The primary fuel source for aerobic activity is body fat and the amount of fat loss due to aerobic movement is directly proportional to the duration and intensity of the activity. In other words, the longer you are able to exercise aerobically, the more your body will turn to your fat stores to fuel your exercise. During the first thirty minutes of aerobic activity, your body will initially obtain its fuel from your muscles and liver. That fuel is in the form of glycogen, which we talked about in Chapter 1. Fortunately for those trying to lose weight, your body has only a limited supply of glycogen available at any one time. So, after the first thirty minutes of a moderate-intensity workout, your body begins using fat as its primary fuel source. Body fat provides virtually an unlimited fuel source, as long as it can be tapped. The key to tapping this energy source is exercising at a moderate intensity for a prolonged period.

The bottom line with aerobic activity is that you need to do at least thirty minutes of this type of exercise to begin burning primarily fat. The longer you work out, the more fat you will burn. The key to extending your aerobic activity to beyond thirty minutes is to keep the intensity moderate.

Reality check: Don't get overwhelmed! This level of activity is your goal. As you will learn in Chapter 7, the process of meeting your fitness goals involves increasing your level of exercise gradually but consistently. If you are able to exercise only for ten minutes at first, that's great! That's ten minutes more than you were doing. Be proud of your accomplishment, but then push yourself a little harder each session. Slowly but surely you will succeed!

Third Tier of the Activity Pyramid: Flexibility and Balance

When you get up in the morning or after sitting for a long time, doesn't it feel great to stretch? Stretching not only feels wonderful, it's important to good fitness. Stretching for flexibility is the most overlooked aspect of an activity program, but it is a crucial one. Don't skip it.

When you exercise, your muscles are forced to stretch beyond their sedentary norm. If these muscles are tight from not having been stretched, they can be easily pulled and even torn. Stretching prepares the muscles for exercise by gently loosening the muscle fibers, thereby increasing their flexibility and reducing your chance of injury.

With increased flexibility from stretching you will:

- Improve your exercise performance.
- Reduce your risk of injury.
- Reduce muscle soreness.
- Improve your posture.
- Reduce low back pain.
- Increase blood flow to the muscle tissues.
- Improve your coordination.
- Reduce stress.
- Enjoy your exercise program more.

When should you stretch? Anytime! However, a warm-up followed by a three-minute to five-minute stretching session will prepare your muscles for the work ahead. But the most important time to stretch is after a workout, because your muscles are warmed up and at their most flexible. Adding stretching to your routine at this point maximizes the range of motion of the muscles you just worked. Think of stretching after a workout as preparation for the next workout. It is also important to learn how to stretch properly, so you do not cause muscle soreness or injury. We will cover that in Chapter 7 "Starting Your Activity Program."

Another neglected aspect of fitness is balance, a capacity that we often take for granted. Older people especially have a generally diminished sense of balance, which is why they are so prone to falls. Practice can help restore this lessened ability. Take children as an example. They naturally practice their balance skills, hopping on one foot, riding a bicycle, or walking over a log. As we get older, however, we tend to gravitate toward activities that do not challenge our sense of balance. Consequently, we begin to lose this innate ability. If your balance is poor, the good news is that you can improve it just like you can improve your muscle strength, flexibility, and aerobic capacity.

Effective exercises for balance include tai chi, yoga, and ballet. But if you do nothing more than practice standing on one foot for a few minutes every day, you will be achieving two goals: expending a few extra calories and keeping your sense of balance alive. So, as part of your regular activity program, try to find a way to hone your balance skills.

Fourth Tier of the Activity Pyramid: Strength Training

Strength training, or resistance training, is as important and perhaps more important to successful fat loss than aerobic exercise. The reason lies in the calories you burn even while you are at rest. By maintaining or building your muscles, you are increasing your calorie-burning potential, even when you are not actually working out.

In one study, subjects on a three-month-long strength training program gained three pounds of muscle and lost four pounds of fat while eating 370 *more* calories per day than they normally did.[10] Aerobic exercise does not increase muscle the way strength training does. Strength training also has been shown to have a positive influence on bone mass.[11]

The good news is that this type of exercise does not have to be done daily to reap its benefits. Just two or three thirty-minute strength training workouts a week is all you need.

In Chapter 7, I will explain in more detail how to strength train, but let me mention here that the most important part of strength training is using proper form. You may want to consider enlisting the help of a fitness trainer to instruct you how to lift weights safely. Many health clubs and gyms offer an initial instruction session for free.

Fifth Tier of the Activity Pyramid: Anaerobic Activity

This type of activity is the kind that really gets your heart pumping. You are doing anaerobic activity when you run to catch a bus, rush across the street before the light changes, or chase after a small child. The key to knowing when you are in an anaerobic mode is that you feel breathless after your exertion.

Obviously, you cannot keep up an anaerobic activity for very long. But the benefits of anaerobic activity for weight loss are huge. This type of exercise has been shown to burn more than three times as much fat as aerobic exercise.[12] However, the combination of anaerobic and aerobic activity results in even faster fat loss than either activity alone.

In small bursts, anaerobic activity revs your engine to exercise at a higher intensity level than you would without it. One way of exercising anaerobically is by interval training. An example of interval training is walking briskly for five minutes, then jogging for one minute, and repeating this for a total time of one hour. Other advantages of anaerobic activity are that it

- can help you to get past a weight-loss plateau.
- increases your aerobic fitness level.
- improves your exercise endurance.
- makes exercise feel easier.
- reduces fatigue from daily activities and increases energy for the day.
- tones the involved muscles.
- adds variety to a perhaps monotonous aerobic routine.

Try to get in some anaerobic activity every week.

Top of the Activity Pyramid: Rest

Ahhhh! After all this talk about moving more, let us not forget the importance of rest. If you exercised every day and never took a break, not only would you possibly burn out, but you could become injured from overusing your muscles. Rest, or recovery, is an *integral* part of any exercise program, especially with strength training, as you must give your muscles a chance to restore themselves after you have worked them hard. Rest will:

- lower lactic acid levels.
- replenish the oxygen in the blood.
- allow your heart rate to return to its resting rate.
- replenish your glycogen stores in the muscles and liver.
- prevent continuous muscle breakdown.
- maintain or improve metabolism.
- improve the productivity of future workouts.

The body's fat-burning potential is maximized when the muscles are allowed to restructure themselves through a combination of exercise and rest. When you are just beginning an exercise program, allow at least one day between workout sessions. As you get in better shape, you can exercise most days, but alternate the type of exercise you do each day. For example, you can do aerobic activity on Mondays, Wednesdays, and Saturdays, and strength and balance training on Tuesdays and Thursdays.

Incorporating Activity into the Wheel of Weight-Management

Each of the four remaining components of the California Wine Country Diet Wheel of Weight-Management—practicality, pleasure, relationships, and variety—is integral to your activity program. Incorporating these components into your physical activities maximizes your chance of long-term success.

Let's take a look at each aspect individually to see how it relates to physical activity.

Practicality

Your activity program must fit practically into your lifestyle if you are going to maintain it over the long term. For one person, going to a health club most days works because childcare is provided. For someone else, the best choice might be heading out the front door for a run because no equipment is involved. Only you can decide what is practical for you.

Pleasure

Even though you may think you cannot possibly derive any pleasure from exercise, think again. One of the known side effects of regular exercise is the release of endorphins, or pleasure hormones, which stimulate a sense of euphoria. Exercising may be uncomfortable at first, but the more you exercise, the more endorphins will be produced and the greater will be your sense of satisfaction and pleasure.

There are other ways you can increase the pleasure of working out. Try exercising to music that provides an uplifting beat to motivate you. You can buy a portable CD player and earphones very inexpensively and make riding that stationary bike a time to catch up on your favorite musician's new release. If you are walking on the treadmill, read that book or magazine that you never find time to read otherwise. With some types of exercise, you can do more than one thing at once—and have fun, too.

Relationships

Social time is a must for many of us, but we often complain that we just do not have the time to keep up with friends and family. Well, there is no reason you cannot use your activity time as a social time. Team up to work out with friends or colleagues, your spouse or significant other, or your kids.

You can use this time to make new friends. If you are out walking in your neighborhood three times a week, sooner or later you will meet the neighbors you never had time to meet before. Or while at the health club you could strike up a conversation with the person on the stationary bike, treadmill, or elliptical machine next to yours. You will find that "shooting the breeze" makes the time speed by—and you might even find that you worked out longer than you usually do. You will no doubt find that your relationships outside of your activity program are also enhanced, for when you feel better about yourself, you feel better about the world and the people you interact with.

Variety

Keeping variety in your activity program is crucial. The enemy of a long-term exercise program is boredom. Avoid lapsing into a routine. Keep your exercise choices interesting, and you will stay interested in exercising. You have myriad types of exercises to choose from and a variety of environments in which to work out, so be creative. By varying your workout, you will not only keep your interest-level high, but you will be doing your body a favor as well because you will be using different sets of muscles, which reduces your chances for soreness or injury. And do not forget to vary the intensity of your activities, perhaps walking one day and upping the intensity with intervals of jogging added to the next day's walk.

Final Food for Thought

Physical activity is important! I know from my own experience and that of hundreds of my clients that the first part of a weight-loss program that gets dropped is exercise. So, it is time for another reality check: You will not sustain any weight loss you do achieve without incorporating an increased level of activity into you daily life. There are simply so many benefits to an increased activity level that it would be a shame not to make it a top priority in your life. With knowledge, a positive attitude, and an adventurous spirit you *can* develop a more active lifestyle. You can not only lose weight, but you can keep it off, increase your fitness, and improve your health. We'll discuss physical activity more in Part II, Chapter 7, "Starting Your Activity Program."

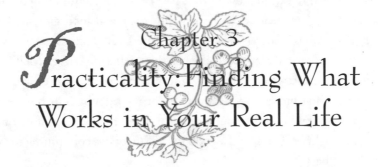

Chapter 3
Practicality: Finding What Works in Your Real Life

"Practical suggests the ability to adapt means to an end..."
—The Random House College Dictionary

Now that we have looked at the basic nutrition and physical activity concepts behind the California Wine Country Diet, it is time to turn our focus to another aspect of the Wheel of Weight-Management that is crucial to long-term success: practicality. No matter how well researched a diet and exercise program may be or how motivated you are, if your plan is not practical, you will not be able to stay with it for very long.

Being *practical*, as the dictionary meaning of this word makes clear, is about choosing means that successfully help you achieve a desired end. The "end" of the California Wine Country Diet is not just weight loss, but a positive change in lifestyle that will ensure long-term weight maintenance and overall health. To reach these goals, you will need to develop practical habits that you can be comfortable with in the years to come.

What is practical varies considerably from person to person, place to place, and time to time. For example, Greek culture, in times past and even today, bears little resemblance to contemporary American culture. As a visitor to Crete in the late 1960s, I remember the serene beauty of this island, which is surrounded by the crystal clear Aegean Sea. At that time, life was very slow moving. Because there were fewer cars, it was necessary for people to walk or take buses. Because people worked close to home, it was practical for them to gather with family for the midday meal and then rest during the hottest part of the day. With limited refrigeration, it was practical to eat fish caught daily and food grown locally. Such a lifestyle is relatively unheard of in the United States today.

In Chapter 1 we looked at the health benefits of Greece's Mediterranean diet. Instinctively we are drawn to the images this diet evokes. Unfortunately that lifestyle is not practical for us. I doubt your boss would agree to your taking three hours off at lunch every day. Even if he or she did, you might have to spend a good part of that time commuting to your home and back.

While you probably cannot return home for lunch with your family every day, there are aspects of the Mediterranean lifestyle you can incorporate into your life. For example, you can make the choice to have home-cooked meals with your family several times each week. While you probably cannot go to a market daily to buy fresh fish or harvest many vegetables you have grown yourself, you can find ways to incorporate fresh, organic, and locally grown produce into your diet.

In the fast-paced world we live in, we have embraced a short-term view of practicality. We look for what saves time and effort each day rather than looking for what is practical in light of our long-term goals. Nowhere can you see this shortsightedness more clearly than in our behaviors surrounding food and physical activity. We eat at drive-thru fast-food restaurants and zap frozen meals to gain a few extra moments in our day. We drive around and around in parking lots to get a space near the door. In the long run, patterns such as these are very impractical, for they have contributed significantly to our national crisis of obesity.

Practicality also applies in less obvious ways. The obesity crisis in our nation affects not only our individual health but also our personal and collective financial health. Researchers from RTI International and the U.S. Department of Health and Human Resources Centers for Disease Control and Prevention estimate that states spend as much as $75 billion a year in medical expenditures related to obesity.[1] Taking time to care for our health makes good financial sense.

Exactly what is practical for you will depend upon your unique style, preferences, and life situation. An important part of the California Wine Country Diet is looking objectively and honestly at yourself so you can develop your own tailor-made plan. As we go along, I will be making suggestions of practical techniques that have worked for many people. It is up to you to select the approaches that you think will work for you, both from my suggestions and from ideas you come up with yourself or glean from other sources. Being willing to try out new things is essential when you are working to change patterns. So let us start with preparing for change.

Practical Preparation

In my book *Choosing to Be Well* readers followed a four-step process that prepared them for taking actions needed to create better health. These four steps of *cooperating, observing, accepting,* and *choosing* will also provide some practical keys for you as you prepare to embark on your weight-loss program. As you can see in the pyramid that follows, in the California Wine Country Diet the four steps come together with a fifth, which I call *conscious indulgence.* I will provide an overview of the steps and then show you how to work with each concept.

The First Tier of the Practicality Pyramid: Cooperating

The different elements of the human psyche have been the subject of study and debate by philosophers over the centuries; now psychologists and neuroscientists have joined the debate. Psychology identifies the conscious self and the unconscious self, or the ego, id, and superego. To keep things simple, I am going to make a distinction between two primary aspects of the self: the conscious self and the basic self. The *conscious self* refers to the voice of the logical, rational mind; whereas the *basic self* refers to the voice of the emotional self, which also is called the child self. These two selves have different styles, skills, and priorities, and it is important that we each learn how we are motivated, controlled, and inspired by our two selves. A major cause of diet failure is the lack of communication between the two selves.

Let us say that you read an article about a diet that makes a strong

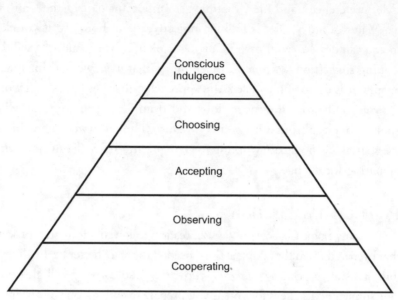

The Practicality Pyramid

impression on your rational self—what we are calling your conscious self—and so you decide to follow that plan. Chances are, if you do so without first consulting your emotional self—what we are calling your basic self—you might find that your success in sticking with the program is short lived. Why? Because your emotional self never agreed to participate and so, sooner or later, will try to sabotage the efforts of your conscious self. You might find yourself feeling unhappy and deprived. You might find yourself obsessing about ice cream or doughnuts—and ultimately giving in. There go your good intentions, and another attempt at dieting fails.

What you need to consider, however, is that it might not have been the ice cream or doughnuts that were so important. Your craving may well have been the call of your basic, emotional self, who was demanding to be heard. The trick to success in changing your nutrition or your activity level—or in just about any other behavior-changing program—is to enlist the aid of both your conscious and your basic selves. If you do not, then in a battle of the wills, the basic self usually wins. We'll get into this a little more later in this chapter.

The Second Tier of the Practicality Pyramid: Observing

The next step in the preparation for any lifestyle change involves looking at how things *really* are—with no excuses, screens, white lies, or diversions, yet with self-compassion and non-judgment. In this step, you train your conscious self to become an objective observer. *Objectivity* means impartially noting what is and not criticizing or blaming yourself for what is.

It is fairly easy to observe with some measure of impartiality the mechanics of our lives—our food choices, our exercise preferences, our work schedules, our hobbies, our personal habits, and so on. But when it comes to observing our physical bodies and our personalities, we face greater challenges. We tend to think we know ourselves, but the truth is that our self-observations are filtered through layers of self-judgment, self-esteem issues, social masks, fears about what we think others think of us, past issues, and the like.

When we observe ourselves from the inside out, we tend to go on the defensive. You know how you blush—or perhaps even cringe—when someone makes a critical comment about you? Well, trust me, you are probably much harder on yourself than anyone else is on you. One problem is that our self-criticisms are not always conscious. That is why learning to observe ourselves through the clear eyes of objectivity, without judgment or condemnation and with compassion and kindness, is crucial to any lifestyle change.

The Third Tier of the Practicality Pyramid: Accepting

Acceptance is the pivotal step that allows us to move on from wherever we are to where we want to be. It means coming to terms with what exists in the present and what has occurred in the past. It means coming to agreement with both your conscious self and your basic self. When you are dealing with weight issues, in particular, achieving acceptance ranges from admitting facts—such as that your metabolism is not working as efficiently as it did when you were in your twenties and so you can no longer eat as much without gaining weight—to facing the lingering emotional effects of far more complicated issues, such as childhood trauma or marital problems.

Addressing these latter issues is beyond the scope of *The California Wine Country Diet*. If you have such issues, you might want to begin examining them in counseling either before starting this program or concurrently, as you undertake it.

Acceptance is often not easy work, but it is crucial to the success of any long-term change. Breaking free from the bonds of denial liberates a wealth of energy to find solutions that will work for you.

The Fourth Tier of the Practicality Pyramid: Choosing

Choosing involves making decisions that will work for the style of your conscious self, the needs of your basic self, and the reality of your life as you have observed it. It is also based on your coming to an acceptance of what is important to you and what you want in your life. Armed with this knowledge, you are better able to motivate yourself not only to make healthy, self-nurturing choices but also to integrate your decisions into your way of being and doing for the long term. Choices made from guilt and feelings of "should" or those based on social pressures and false ideals are choices that are doomed to failure. In contrast, clear-cut and informed decisions tend to motivate you and increase your chances for success. All your actions are based on choice, so it is crucial to make sure you know why you are choosing what you are.

Top of the Practicality Pyramid: Conscious Indulgence

Conscious indulgence is at the heart of successfully incorporating the California Wine Country Diet program into your daily life. It is a concept that integrates the logical wisdom of your conscious self and the innate insight of your basic self. Conscious indulgence is the key that will allow you to enjoy the pleasures of life while remaining attentive to its practical requirements. Especially as you age, maintaining a healthy weight requires being conscious of what you eat and how much you exercise. Yet if you do not "indulge" in what gives you pleasure, rebellion will soon set in.

In the California Wine Country Diet, you will be practicing conscious indulgence from the first day of the diet. Since structure is very important when learning new patterns, you will be given daily food plans for the first three weeks. You will also have a certain number of calories each day for "wine and other pleasures." This is where you will begin practicing the art of conscious indulgence. Remember the saying that "the price of freedom is eternal vigilance"? In the California Wine Country Diet, your price is the vigilance of being conscious. Your reward is good health, freedom from a life of yo-yo dieting, and the joys of the table.

More About the Practicality Pyramid

Each of these five tiers of the practicality pyramid is crucial to finding a realistic, and hence successful, personal program for achieving your goal. These are not steps you take once and then have mastered. You will find yourself coming back to each of them again and again as your life situation changes, as you grow and change as a human being, and as you face new goals or challenges. Different people find different tiers, or steps, of the pyramid easier—or harder—to negotiate. This is why tier 2, "Observing," is so crucial not only as you begin this program but over the long term. Observation helps get you on track to make decisions about what you want to change. But you also must remain observant throughout the entire process, so that you can identify stumbling blocks and understand how to overcome them. For instance, it is by being impartially observant that you will be able to determine if you are continuing to "cooperate" (tier 1) and if you are "choosing" well (tier 4). Very simply, without good observation skills, you cannot monitor your progress well—and truthfully—and so cannot adjust your course if necessary.

We each have different strengths and weaknesses, and if we observe ourselves impartially and with compassion, we can admit that a stumbling block does not have to be a roadblock to our success. It simply requires more of our attention.

Let me provide a couple of real-life examples from my psychotherapy practice about how following the steps—or not—can affect success or failure. I would like to point out, first, that the best way to achieve success is to remember that this program is not a weight-loss program primarily, but a *lifestyle* program. So, as you read each example, be aware of how easy it is to slip back into the "old model" of dieting for a while and then returning to your old habits. Pay attention to how shifting to the "new model"—by keeping in mind the California Wine Country Diet program, and the practicality pyramid in particular—can help you move toward success.

For "Susan," the struggle came in maintaining cooperation between her rational, conscious self and her more emotional basic self (tier 1). After successfully reaching her goal weight, she continued to prepare or choose healthy foods when she was by herself. But when she was with her friends, she was unable to resist the foods they tended to order or prepare—large quantities of fried foods and desserts. Susan was fully aware of this conflict, so she was observant of her behavior (tier 2), but she could not seem to control the outcome of the battle within. Rationally, she fully understood that when she was in these kinds of social situations, she had the power of choice about what to eat and how much, but her basic self seemed to take control, protesting, "I should be able to eat whatever they're eating." Her basic self always won. Susan's ability to choose (tier 4) was compromised. The divide between her conscious self and her basic self signaled deeper work that Susan had to do about social acceptance and other personal issues. But the fact that she would not accept (tier 3) that if she was going to maintain her weight loss she could not eat the same way her friends ate led to a failure of choice (tier 4).

"Tom" faithfully followed a sensible eating plan and found many new physical activities that he enjoyed, but as soon as he had reached his weight-loss goal, he decided to become more "unconsciously indulgent" (tier 5). Basically, he began to add back some of his favorite foods, such as potato chips and chocolate chip cookies, which had always led him to compulsive and unconscious eating in the past. He also stopped weighing himself. Over time, he began to notice that the waistband of his pants was feeling snugger, but conveniently ignored this clue that he was regaining the weight he had lost. Because Tom chose not to "accept" (tier 3) his observation (tier 2), he did not change or modify his behavior and soon he had regained all the weight he had lost. For Tom, his first challenge was in choosing to abandon the parameters of the conscious indulgence tier. Then his primary challenges shifted to tiers 2 and 3 of the practicality pyramid—observing and accepting. While he was happy to observe how he lost weight, he went into denial as the weight began to come back on, and he chose to deny that his food choices—or the quantity of those foods he was indulging in—were the cause. But if Tom had truly observed the signs and then accepted them at face value, he could have made a few small changes in following tier 5 that would have put him back on track.

Susan and Tom certainly are not alone in their struggle with food and weight. Studies show that most people regain two-thirds of the weight they lose on diets within a year and almost all the weight they lost within five years.[2] The underlying problem is that diets are rarely long-term programs for choosing a healthy lifestyle. They are short-term fixes. This is where the California Wine Country Diet is different. Your goal is not only to lose weight, but to adopt a healthy and nurturing lifestyle. More important, it is about doing all this while also making choices that fulfill your need for pleasure and satisfaction. With the California Wine Country Diet, you should not have to struggle, as Susan did, with reconciling your conscious self and your more emotional basic self. You will learn how to satisfy them both through conscious indulgence.

The steps that I have outlined above are crucial to any long-term change. So, let's continue to use them to explore your personal style, your potential stumbling blocks, and what choices are truly practical in your life. Consider the following questions. Write your answers on a sheet of paper. Be as truthful and impartial as you can.

Tier 1 — Cooperating

- What does your conscious self think about starting the California Wine Country Diet program?
- What does your basic self feel about starting the California Wine Country Diet program?
- Where are your conscious self and your basic self in disagreement or conflict?
- What compromises can your conscious and basic selves make that would satisfy each of their concerns and/or needs?

Tier 2 — Observing

Home Environment

- Do you have a bathroom scale in good working order for weighing yourself weekly during weight loss and more frequently during maintenance?

- As objectively as you can, describe the physical space where you prepare and/or eat the majority of your meals.

- How does that space make you feel?

- What is pleasing about that space?

- What is not so pleasing about it?

- Do you have the proper equipment (pots, pans, utensils, etc.) to make cooking at home easy and enjoyable?

- How does your overall physical home environment (uncluttered counters and table tops, noise levels, comfort levels, relaxing atmosphere, privacy issues, and such) support your desire to lose weight and have a healthier lifestyle? How does it challenge that goal?

- How would you say your present home responsibilities support your desire to lose weight and begin living a healthier lifestyle? How do they challenge that goal?

- Do you eat on a regular basis or schedule with your family, roommates, or other persons you live with, or are you and they on a hectic or varied schedule?

- What are the potential challenges or supportive features of that eating schedule?

- If you live with others, what is the role of each person in food purchasing, preparation, and clean up? Will the other members of your household be eating the foods of the California Wine Country Diet? If not, how will you accommodate that?

- What are some of the other ways your personal relationships at home support or hamper your lifestyle-change goal?

- When will you take time to select your food plans for the week? How often will you shop?

Work Environment

- How does your work schedule currently contribute to your weight and fitness problems?

- What time do you have to get up?

- Do you eat breakfast?

- How long is your commute? Do you eat in the car or on the train?

- What is the food environment like where you work?

- Is there a lunchroom or break room where snacks and sodas are kept? How often do you visit it?

- Do you take a lunch break or eat at your desk?

- Is there a refrigerator for food you bring to work? A microwave for heating food you bring?

- Are your coworkers health conscious? Do they walk or exercise during the workday?

- What is your level of stress during the workday?

- Do you eat when you get stressed at work?

Lifestyle and Social Environment

- How often do you eat at restaurants?

- What type of restaurant do you most often frequent—a sit-down, full-menu restaurant, or take-out or fast food restaurants?

- How does eating at this type of restaurant support your weight-loss program and desire for a healthier lifestyle? How does it challenge it?

- How does eating in the homes of others support your weight-loss and lifestyle goal? How does this challenge it?

- How often do you "eat on the run"? What do you usually eat in this circumstance?

Rating Your Lifestyle

As an objective and nonjudgmental observer, rate your overall present lifestyle as it pertains to your diet on a scale of 1 to 10. A score of 1 equals a not at all health-promoting lifestyle, and a score of 10 signifies a highly health-promoting lifestyle. What did you give yourself? Are you satisfied with this score? Now do the same thing in the area of physical activity. Are you satisfied?

Tier 3 — Accepting

Look back at your answers to the questions in "Tier 2—Observing." You have accumulated a wealth of information about the three primary areas of your life: home, work, and social/life style. As you review your answers, consider the following questions:

- Do you notice any patterns or trends?

- What are your areas of greatest support?

- What are your areas of greatest challenge?

- From whom and how can you get more support?

- Do you need professional support for certain problems or challenges?

Acceptance means that you are aware of the issue and able to assume responsibility for it. To determine if you really accept the reality of your situation, think of your feelings as you considered an area. Did you feel angry? Sad? Ashamed? Confused? If so, make note of these feelings because they point to areas where you were in a state of resistance, not acceptance. If you have identified an area of resistance, ask yourself if you can imagine a solution to the problem or somehow otherwise imagine the situation resolving itself so that you can impartially accept it.

As an example, suppose that you observe that you eat out a lot because you do not like to cook. As you consider that statement, you notice that you feel a bit uneasy, even a little bit ashamed. You do not really accept it. So you examine your vague emotions without judgment and discover that this is not really a true observation. You eat out a lot not because you do not like to cook but because you are usually too tired to cook when you get home from work. That makes you feel a little guilty because you know, if you cooked, you (and perhaps your family) might eat healthier food. When you can accept this observation as truth—and the tinge of guilt that goes with it—then there is no longer any emotional conflict around it. You own the observation and accept how it makes you feel.

To help you come to acceptance around areas that might be causing you discomfort and to find solutions, use the question below. However, make sure you answer it based on the *real* observation, not the assumed one. Also, do not limit yourself to one short answer. If other associations, ramifications, insights, or solutions present themselves, write them down as well. Before you begin, let me provide an example:

Question: What do I need to accept about my (home environment, work environment, lifestyle) in order to be successful at weight loss and weight management?

Answer: What I need to accept about my lifestyle in order to be successful at weight loss and weight management is that I will not be preparing a lot of my own meals as long as I stay in my current job unless I find a way to prepare meals ahead of time (like on the weekends). I'm just too tired at the end of the day. This means I have to make better choices about where I eat (not fast-food places) and what I choose to eat. I'll probably also have to watch portion size, as restaurants today tend to serve oversized portions.

Now it's your turn. Complete the following sentence as it pertains overall to each of the three primary areas of your life.

What I need to accept about my (home environment, work environment, lifestyle) in order to be successful at weight loss and weight management is _____.

Tier 4 — Choosing

You are now ready to make practical choices in the three main areas of your life that will help you succeed with the California Wine Country Diet program. As you select techniques for dealing with challenging situations, evaluate your choices, and make sure that they feel right emotionally. As you go through each area, I will make suggestions. Make a note of those that you want to try. Then come up with additional ideas of your own. Be sure to keep adding to your lists as you discover new ideas.

Practical Keys for Your Home Environment

Your home is the foundation for your new way of eating even if you eat out several times a week. In the process of clearing out and organizing your physical environment, you will also be preparing yourself for changes in your daily patterns.

- Sit down with those who live in your house and tell them about starting the California Wine Country Diet. Ask for the specific types of support you would like from them. Invite them to join you in this new way of eating.

- Clean out your kitchen cupboards to get ready for starting the program. Throw out, give away, or put safely away all foods that tempt you to overeat. It is often helpful to remove everything and then put back only those food items that support the program.

- Begin the practice of measuring or weighing everything you eat and looking at serving sizes for calorie amounts on food containers. Eventually you will be able to judge by eyeing quantities. We will not use the term "portion control" since it tends to bring up feelings of rebellion against "controlling authority." Through conscious indulgence you will be keeping an eye on amounts while eating the foods you love.

- Have a collection of measuring utensils conveniently at hand: multiple sets of measuring spoons, several measuring cups, and a convenient food scale. This way you will have no excuse for not weighing and measuring your food.

- Have a collection of storage containers for extra portions and for food you will take to work.

- Avoid second helpings by putting away extra food immediately. Enjoy these foods as "more indulgence" the next day. What a great way to combine practicality and pleasure!

- Gather or buy small plates and tall thin glasses. Both give the illusion of having more.

- Keep a basket of fresh fruit on the counter to encourage the eating of these healthy foods.

- Establish a consistent time each week when you will evaluate the past week and make menu plans for the coming week. You can make copies of the Daily Meal Plan in Chapter 9 or you can download a copy at www.CaliforniaWineCountryDiet.com. Keep the forms you fill out for review and for future planning.

- Based on your menu plans, draw up a shopping list.

- Shop once or twice a week from a list to avoid impulse buying.

- Shop at your local farmers' market or co-op to encourage eating fresh, locally grown produce. (This also is a wonderful social experience and supports small farmers.)

- Review your Daily Meal Plan each night. Check to see that you have eaten the recommended servings in each category, and rate how you have attended to the six aspects of weight management by using the "Five-Star Rating System" on the form. While you are losing weight and developing new habits, you will need to give your meal plan closer attention to than you will later on when the habit has become second nature.

Now make a list of your own ideas.

Practical Keys for Your Work Environment

It is extremely difficult to lose or maintain weight if you are only eating the foods available at workplaces and restaurants. You must plan ahead and bring food from home whenever you can.

- Plan for each work day, knowing what you will be taking from home for lunch and for snacks.

- Make sure you always bring two healthy snacks with you to avoid spur-of-the-moment, high-calorie snacks.

- Eat the second snack before you leave work so you will not overeat when you get home.

- Always have plenty of water and other healthy beverages, such as green tea, on hand.

- Avoid skipping meals, and eat at scheduled times so that you don't get too hungry.

- Always have some emergency food (can of tuna fish, nuts) in your desk drawer or locker so that you are never in a position of getting hungry and having to eat out of the vending machine.

- Avoid locations where high-calorie food is left out for nibbling.

- Refuse to bend to pressure from others to eat. If possible, ask for their support.

- Use part of your lunch time for exercise.

- Find colleagues who are also eating healthy foods and support each other.

- If you are going to eat out with coworkers make sure that you go to a restaurant that will have food choices compatible with your new, healthier lifestyle.

Now make a list of your ideas.

Practical Keys for Your Social Environment

Visiting friends, going out to dinner or a movie, attending a sporting event—these are all situations where it is easy to surrender control over your food choices. By planning ahead and not being afraid to ask for what you want, you can find ways to enjoy yourself and still keep on track with your eating plan.

Here are some ideas for dealing with social situations:

- When you are invited to eat at someone's home, ask if you can bring a dish. Then bring a large green or fruit salad that you can fill up on, depending on what else is served.

- Eat before going so that you are not too hungry, especially at events that will have lots of nibble food.

- In restaurants, ask for what you want. Inquire about how entrees are prepared, and request heavy sauces be omitted from a dish. Ask for an extra serving of vegetables or fruit to replace fried potatoes or other high-calorie choices.

- Always ask for salad dressing to be put on the side.

- Eat smaller amounts. Since restaurants often serve large portions, try different approaches to eating less. You can divide an entree, order an appetizer, or put aside part of your meal to take home.

- Practice the art of leaving something on your plate.

- Never leave home without taking a bottle of water with you.

- Never leave home for more than an hour without taking a healthy snack with you.

List some of your own ideas.

Getting Started

You may be feeling quite overwhelmed with all the ideas presented in this chapter. Take a few deep breaths and remember that health is a life-long process. You have identified a lot of choices you can make to begin eating better and living a healthier life. Choose a few that most excite you or seem easiest or that are most in sync with your current circumstances. Remember that you are just getting started and that you will implement this program gradually.

One suggestion for getting started is to begin evaluating the contents of your kitchen and cleaning out what no longer serves you in your new, healthier goals. If you work on this clearing-out process while you are reading through the next three chapters of Part I, you will be ready to go by the time you reach Part II and the actual eating plan.

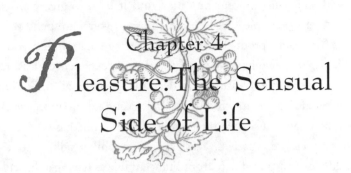

Chapter 4
Pleasure: The Sensual Side of Life

Pleasure—The gratification of the senses or of the mind;
agreeable sensations or emotions; the excitement, relish or
happiness produced by the expectation or the enjoyment
of something good, delightful, or satisfying...
—Webster's Revised Unabridged Dictionary, 1913

As we move from the logical sphere of practicality to the sensual realm of pleasure, take a moment to imagine that you are sitting in front of a crackling fire, sipping a glass of Merlot or Port, and savoring a piece of rich dark chocolate. Ah, pleasure! Just let the silky tones of the word "pleasure" roll off your tongue. How very different from the hard-edged sound of "practical."

With an eye to building on the foundation laid in the first three chapters of *The California Wine Country Diet*—nutrition, physical activity, and practicality—let's now turn our attention to what gives you pleasure and how you can satisfy your palate while both losing weight and maintaining that weight loss.

From the very beginning of life, food and drink have been among our greatest pleasures. Depending on our experiences in childhood and the rest of our life, our innate ability to relish pleasure has either been nurtured or stifled. In addition to the attitudes and practices we learned from our families, we soon encountered the popular view that eating that which gives us pleasure is somehow spoiling ourselves or at least is bad for our health. So, while you might think that pleasure would be the easiest of all the six aspects to embrace, it is not. In fact, for many readers it will be the most difficult.

Those of you who have spent a lifetime dieting or who are struggling with compulsive overeating may find it hard to give yourself permission to enjoy the pleasure of food. Those of you who spend your days rushing from one "productive activity" to another may find your difficulty lies in actually giving yourself the time to experience pleasure.

Our aversion to pleasure runs deep in our national spirit. While we in the United States come from just about every culture in the world, the Puritan heritage that shaped the American work ethic has set the scale by which we measure ourselves. Years ago, I remember talking to a friend who had recently moved here from France. He was having a difficult time adjusting to how the American mindset seemed fixated on business. He said that in France, when friends gathered at parties, they talked about food, wine, and life, whereas, in the United States, people talked mostly about their work life.

The average American is working one month (160 hours) more each year than a generation ago.[1] We eat at our desks or in our car to save time for more work. By the time vacation rolls around, we are often too exhausted to enjoy it. In addition to working longer hours, with both spouses working, there is the second job at the end of the day—taking care of family and home. On top of all that is the deluge bombarding us from television, newspapers, e-mail, and the Internet. Who has time in all of this whirlwind to think about pleasure?

Our ambivalence about pleasure is perhaps most clearly evident in our attitude toward food. The eating disorders of anorexia nervosa and bulimia represent the extreme ends of our dieting culture. Both of these eating disorders usually begin with dieting and the desire to exceed our cultural imperative to be thin. The anorexic person begins her quest for perfection by restricting intake, but eventually reaches a point where she feels guilty about eating anything at all. The bulimic person rebels against restriction with secretive binge eating followed by purging, restricting food intake, or undertaking a regime of excessive exercise to maintain normal weight.

Although the majority of us are not suffering from medically diagnosed eating-disorders, huge numbers of us are obsessed with our diet. *The Random House Webster's College Dictionary's* definition of diet is "food considered in terms of its qualities, composition, and effects on health."[2] As a society, however, we have narrowed the meaning of this word to "trying to lose weight." The emphasis is on the word "trying." As we have talked about earlier in the book, we have become a culture of yo-yo dieters, caught in a vicious cycle of gaining weight, feeling bad about ourselves and feeling guilty for our overeating, and then radically changing the way we eat—and consequently the way we feel—in an effort to lose the excess pounds.

The truth is that this kind of weight-gain, weight-loss cycle is not really about food at all. It is more about how we are failing to satisfy ourselves in a healthy, sustainable way. We fall almost unconsciously into a cycle of pleasure-punishment and self-gratification-self-denial.

In the dieting process, we forgo the foods we love in order to lose weight, but we eventually are driven by emotional and physical feelings of deprivation back to our favorite treats. How do we stop this cycle and bring a measure of sanity back into our culinary and emotional lives? By not denying ourselves pleasure in the first place.

While we fear that pleasure is the demon causing our weight gain, it is not. Let me repeat that: *Pleasure is not your enemy!* But not understanding what brings you pleasure can be a problem. For most people, the greatest pleasure in eating and drinking comes in the first few tastes. Our added pounds result from continuing to eat beyond either our pleasure quotient or our appetite. Instead, we are driven by unconscious, compulsive patterns. Just as you learned to look at practicality through a long-term lens in Chapter 3, so will you now begin to look at finding long-term pleasure in every aspect of your experience with food: from the anticipation of a good meal, to the appreciation of it, to the satisfaction of having eaten food in an amount that agrees with your body.

Embrace the Pleasure

One of the fundamental principles of the California Wine Country Diet program is that you must give yourself permission to let go of any punitive attitudes you may have toward enjoying food. It is time to give yourself permission to not feel guilty about your love of food by learning to embrace conscious indulgence. By understanding and welcoming the pleasure you find in eating, you can begin to make real and permanent strides toward achieving and maintaining a healthy weight, good health, and a more satisfying lifestyle.

Pleasure and the Basic Self

The term *hedonics* refers to the branch of psychology that deals with pleasurable and unpleasurable states of consciousness. It comes from the Greek word *hedon*, which means "pleasure," a subject that has been a focus of philosophers, psychologists, and scientists since the time of ancient Greece. At the turn of the twentieth century, the prevailing theory was that the main forces that motivate us are the simple processes of approaching pleasant stimuli and avoiding painful stimuli.[3]

But actually there is nothing simple about such a pleasure-pain process. Today, research shows that the pleasure systems of the brain are extremely complex, and the perception of pleasure plays a part in most of our decision making. "Pleasure helps us plan our movements and allows our brains to filter and sort out the mass of smells, sights, sounds, and other information that bombard our senses."[4]

Researcher Helen Phillips from the University of Wisconsin, Madison, believes that only when we fully understand the brain's pleasure and desire circuits are we "likely to make progress in understanding two of the biggest threats to public health in the developed world, obesity and drug addiction."[5]

While neuroscience continues to investigate the complex systems of the human brain, what we know at this point is very helpful in understanding the important role of pleasure in maintaining weight. First of all, we understand now that pleasure is an inborn mechanism that is necessary for our survival. The positive sensations we anticipate and then experience motivate us to eat and drink. Pleasure has natural limits and ends when our need is fulfilled. Pleasure guides us in knowing when we have had enough. It can guide us to the foods that are best for us by providing feedback on how our bodies feel after we have eaten. The bottom line is that we need not fear pleasure. It is not only a necessity; it is one of life's greatest joys.

Moreover, we could say that the pleasure centers of our brain are the domain of our basic self. The basic self, as explained earlier, is our emotional center. Some call it our child self. It stands in contrast to our rational, analytical, logical, conscious self. What happens in so many dieting situations is that we totally abandon our responsibility to our basic self. We diet by depriving ourselves, thus abandoning the sensory delights our basic self thrives on. When the basic self finally erupts in protest, then we "cheat" on our diet or abandon it all together. What we need to realize is that our basic self is indeed like an unruly child that we have to love while exerting a measure of control over. Like good parents, we need to listen to the needs of our child without letting him or her run our lives.

Our adult role in weight management is to listen to the pleasure signals of our bodies, while also gathering nutritional information, and then setting guidelines that will be in our best interest. Our basic self has strong opinions about what it likes and does not like—your basic self might love chocolate, while mine loves ice cream. We can indulge our truly basic likes and dislikes while still losing weight. The rest of this chapter talks about finding the pleasure in eating by honoring the basic self without allowing it to control us.

Pleasure and Weight Management

Giving the basic self free rein can result in overeating (as in binge eating), as can denying the basic self any say whatsoever in our food choices (the usual diet mind-set and its corresponding sense of deprivation). I have found the work of writer and teacher Geneen Roth invaluable in understanding the psychological causes of compulsive overeating. Some years ago I attended one of her seminars for therapists in San Francisco. At the lunch break, we were given instructions to find a restaurant where we could eat "what we really wanted to eat." Finding a mutually agreeable lunch spot for any group of strangers is difficult, much less a group of therapists who had been given the above instructions in a city with some of the best restaurants in the world.

It is surprising that any of us ate lunch that day, as we wandered in and out of restaurants trying to decide on the cuisine that truly satisfied our desires. We were searching not for what was *convenient*, but for what we *really wanted*.

Just by posing the question to myself I learned that what I usually eat may not be what I want, but rather what is most readily available, or the preference of my companions or what I think I should eat. Through such self-analysis, I learned a valuable lesson that day. I discovered how difficult it is to know what I truly wanted—and then how it is even more difficult to give myself permission to have it.

Roth's program is built on the belief that if we eat what we *really* want and eat *only* until we are satisfied, we will not overeat. While this sounds simple, it is a challenge for those who choose what they eat based on a plethora of reasons that have nothing to do with personal food preference. These reasons often include pleasing others, boredom, emotional pain, and anger. Allowing yourself to have the foods you truly love can at first be a frightening experience. After that, it is exhilarating.

In reviewing Roth's "Eating Guidelines," I was delighted to see how well they fit with the California Wine Country Diet philosophy and specifically with the role pleasure plays in weight management. Her guidelines recommend the following: Eat when you are hungry, eat sitting down in a calm environment, eat without distraction, eat only what you want, eat until you are satisfied, and eat with enjoyment, pleasure, and gusto.[6]

Keep these guidelines in mind throughout the rest of this chapter—and indeed the rest of this book. These are pillars of any long-term weight-loss and weight-management program. Let us now look at different aspects of "pleasure" by exploring the California Wine Country Diet pleasure pyramid.

The First Tier of the Pleasure Pyramid: Taking Time and Slowing Down

Time and pleasure are almost synonymous. Try to imagine truly enjoying a meal that you have rushed through. It is not possible, because pleasure requires focus and focus requires a slowing down of activity. Think about experiences that you have truly enjoyed, about the weekends and vacations that are cherished memories. A large part of what makes vacations so refreshing is that in stepping away from the rush of our daily lives time seems to slow down so that all our senses are heightened.

Remember the research mentioned in Chapter 3 that examined the

Mediterranean diet and physical activities of the people living on the Greek island of Crete in the 1960s? Nancy Harmon Jenkins, author of *The Mediterranean Diet Cookbook*, suggests the need for research into other lifestyle factors as well which may have greatly contributed to the residents' good health. She includes in this list "the extensive amount of time spent relaxing over meals, offering a relief from daily stress" and "the post-lunch tradition of siesta (a good, long afternoon nap) that also provides relief from stress."[7] At that time, most people came home at midday for a leisurely lunch, which was the main meal of the day. After lunch, in the hottest part of the day, people took a long rest or nap before returning to work. What a wonderful way to live. Imagine being able to sleep when that mid-afternoon doziness hits you, rather than trying to pump yourself up with cups of coffee to make it through the work day.

Across the planet there is a growing consciousness that the speed of our modern world is threatening our physical and emotional health, both individually and collectively. The Slow Food Movement is one response

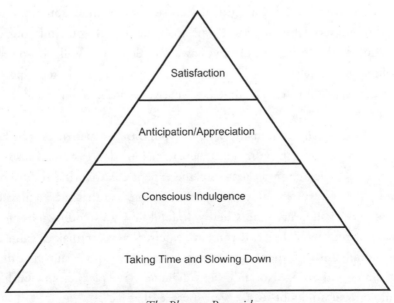

The Pleasure Pyramid

to the increasing worldwide proliferation of the fast-food eating trend and its negative health consequences. Founded by Carlo Petrini in Italy in 1986, this nonprofit organization is now active in forty-five countries. Its focus is to preserve food varieties that were being annihilated and cultural food traditions that were disappearing. The Slow Food Movement believes that pleasure and quality of life are achieved by slowing down and enjoying food in the context of convivial relationships. For more information on the activities of this organization go to www.slowfoodusa.org.

While most dieticians would recommend having your largest meal at midday, and it is obvious that we would benefit from taking time to rest, in today's hubbub-filled world, there are very few who could change their lifestyle to do this. The time you find for pleasure will have to be within the real-life schedule you keep. And the truth is, finding pleasure in your normally hectic schedule may require a perceptual shift on your part—a change in the way you think.

Here are some fundamental ideas for slowing down and enjoying your body, diet, and life. You can come up with other ideas for increasing the pleasure in your life that are realistic for your particular situation and schedule.

For most of us, it is most realistic to begin making small changes, and then to add additional new behaviors slowly over time. You can begin by finding moments of "down time" in your day. If you find yourself rushing to the office, try to slow down and enjoy the walk. If you are talking on the telephone to a colleague or friend, try really focusing on the conversation instead of thinking what you will be doing the minute you hang up the phone.

Be especially mindful in relation to your dining experiences, whether a morning snack at the office or dinner after a long day. Instead of rushing through a snack or meal, draw out the experience, savoring the flavors and pleasing textures of the food you are eating. Sip that special glass of wine over a half hour's time. Chew your food slowly, extending the enjoyment of your food choice. If you have children, you can make a game of being mindful with them, so that they will learn to appreciate what they are doing and eating. Not only will you increase the pleasure in your life, but you will no doubt reduce your stress level as well.

The Second Tier of the Pleasure Pyramid: Conscious Indulgence

The next level on the pleasure pyramid is conscious indulgence. This is where you choose to indulge in any food you find pleasurable. But indulge within reason.

When it comes to heightening your enjoyment of eating and drinking, while still managing your weight, one of the most important perceptual shifts is to bring awareness to portion size. In Part II, you will be counselled to take the time to weigh and measure your food portions when you can, at least as you begin the program. I will also suggest visual cues to help you estimate portion sizes when you cannot weigh and measure, such as when dining out.

While it takes a few extra minutes to do so, managing your portion size is a worthy trade-off for allowing yourself to eat what you really want. Realistically, which option would you choose: Eating what you really like every day, but in measured quantities? Or, eating bigger portions of what you really do not want every day but what you think is "good for you"? To be more concrete, which is more desirable for you: a pre-measured slice of chocolate cake or a store-bought bag of mini carrots? When you think in the long term, the choice is obvious.

There are some visual tricks that can be very useful in limiting portion size while fulfilling your "pleasure perception." Drinking from a tall, thin glass has been found to create a sense of having more to drink than drinking the same amount from a short, round glass.

The same idea works with plates and dishes. You can purchase some small plates on which to serve snacks, or what the Greeks call *meze*. (To increase your pleasure quotient, indulge in a few exquisite plates.) I use this trick myself. I recently bought some five-inch-diameter, hand-painted dishes. It is amazing how pleasurable it is to eat off a beautiful small plate. At times I pile my whole lunch onto a small plate and it feels like I am having a giant feast simply because the plate is overflowing. Having been raised to be a member of the "Clean your plate club," I enjoy the comfort of finishing everything on my plate.

When you are first beginning to pay more attention to your portion size, it will be important to measure what you are eating according to the menu plans and recipes presented in Part II. Be sure to have a food scale, several measuring cups, and a variety of measuring spoons conveniently at hand. At home you can begin to estimate portions by how they look on your familiar dishes or in your glasses. Finally, you will begin to estimate portions by the size of the helping.

It helps to discipline yourself to limit portions by cutting meats or other foods into standard-size servings and packaging them individually for refrigeration or freezing. That way you can take out only what you need. Also, take the time to read the serving-size recommendations on packaged food. How many suggested servings does each package contain? Do you follow that recommendation? If not, try to follow it next time you prepare it.

In Chapter 9, you will learn about specific standard-serving sizes and methods for estimating portions. To begin, just allow this valuable principle to work its way into your perceptual habits so that your basic self will be in agreement with practicing conscious indulgence when you begin the actual menu plans of the California Wine Country Diet. Shift your mind-set now, and more conscious behavioral changes will come more easily later.

Conscious Indulgence Exercise

There are many creative ways to reduce portion size and follow portion recommendations. The paragraphs above discussed some ideas. Now it is your turn to think creatively. Take a piece of paper and make a list of the foods and beverages that give you the greatest pleasure. Put an X next to those that challenge you the most in limiting your portions.

Now write down all the ways you can eat what gives you pleasure but in conscious amounts. Try to keep your basic self in mind, so that you can fulfill the needs of both your pleasure-seeking self and your more conscious, rational, health-conscious self.

For instance, if you love chocolate bars, perhaps you could break one up into small squares, wrap each "serving" in foil, and store these individual portions in a zip lock bag. That way you can still eat what you love, but you will be less tempted later to open the whole bar and eat it at one sitting. You also could brainstorm "prompts" that will help you remember to eat each "serving" in a lingering way and so truly enjoy it. For instance, you could repeat a phrase in your mind between each bite: "Slow down, savor, and enjoy."

Once you have brainstormed ideas, circle those you think are most brilliant (and practical) and put them into use immediately. There may be foods which you compulsively overeat and conscious indulgence with them is not realistic at this point. We will look further at what to do about these foods in Chapter 11.

The Third Tier of the Pleasure Pyramid: Anticipation/Appreciation

We look forward to those things that bring us pleasure. Eating is certainly one of them. But what is missing from many people's dining experience is the pleasure of the *anticipation* of eating, especially when it comes to eating at home.

What makes eating out so pleasurable? For most of us, it is taking our time to enjoy the experience without other distractions, savoring the atmosphere, and admiring the presentation of the meal on the plate. These are all *sensory aspects* of the dining environment that you have control over right in your own home. But most of us ignore them. We think they are not important. But they are, and we should use them to our advantage.

Anticipation often begins with a perceptual change that happens long before you sit down to eat. For instance, what is your perception of food preparation? For most of us it is a chore. It is usually just one more thing that has to be done at the end of a long day of work before we can relax. What would happen to your mood, however, if you considered food preparation as an opportunity to indulge your senses and your sense of service to yourself and others? One shift of perception can make all the difference in whether you find pleasure or pain in the moment.

So, how could you make that shift? Perhaps as you make up your weekly menus, you could take time to look through mouth-watering pictures in cookbooks. You could talk to your family about what they want to eat in the coming days with the anticipation of knowing your efforts will bring them and you pleasure. As you shop, you could decide to be appreciative of the plethora of choices you have before you. You could decide to be attentive to the textures of the vegetables, the colors of the packaging, the incredible array of sensory cues that are competing for your attention.

Advertisers certainly know the value of visual and other sensory cues in attracting you to their foods. In photo ads, a steak has perfectly aligned grill marks, and it is cut open to show you its tender, juicy, pink inside. In TV ads, potato chips crunch and bowls of soup give off enticing wisps of steam. You get the idea. And it is one worth keeping in mind as you find ways to increase the sensory pleasure of the meals you prepare at home.

There is a myriad of other ways to increase your anticipation of pleasurable food moments. They all require your *intention* to find the pleasure in the moment and your *attention* to your experience. Instead of "throwing something together" for dinner (or breakfast or lunch), consciously decide to "prepare" dinner. It usually does not take any more time to do something well than to do it sloppily.

Anticipating and appreciating your dining experience starts not with the act of eating but with the intention of creating a "dining experience." As you actually prepare food, take the initiative to make it appealing—even beautiful. Arrange the food pleasingly, using a sprig of parsley or a slice of lemon to dress up the plate. Indulge your creativity.

Create a pleasant atmosphere as well. Instead of using the everyday plates, use the good china you usually save for special occasions. Dress the table with a colorful tablecloth, a vase of fresh flowers, some artfully placed candles. Then turn off the television (!) and put on some nice dinner music.

As you sit down to your meal, do not forget to indulge all of your senses. Take a moment to appreciate the food that is before you by looking at it, smelling it, even admiring it. Give thanks for it. Then take a taste of each different kind of food on your plate and allow its taste to linger and its smell to satisfy. Revel in the results of your mindful effort in preparing the food. Plan for the dinner to be special and it will be.

Although these ideas are concentrated around a main meal eaten at home, learn to anticipate and appreciate every meal, no matter where it is eaten or what you are eating.

Anticipation/Appreciation Exercise

Anticipation involves "active imagination." Try sitting quietly and imagining what a perfect meal would be like. What is the atmosphere? The location? The lighting? Whom are you with? How is the table prepared? How do you feel? Visualize an appetizing, beautifully presented meal of healthy food. See yourself eating it—and enjoying it, slowly and appreciatively. See yourself eating only until you are satisfied, which may not be the same thing as "until you are full." Congratulate yourself on eating healthily and with pleasure.

Then brainstorm how you can make your usual eating area (for instance, your home kitchen or dining room) more pleasurable. Atmosphere has everything to do with anticipation and sensory pleasure. Imagine how you can present the food you cook more appealingly. If you cannot think of ways to make your everyday dining experiences more pleasurable, go to the library and look at decorating and cookbooks for ideas about how to make your room more attractive or how to present food artfully.

The Fourth Tier of the Pleasure Pyramid: Satisfaction

Long-term weight loss and weight management are absolutely dependent on your sensory satisfaction. Very simply, how you eat, what you eat, and how much you eat has to be pleasurable and satisfying—enough to motivate you to make your new eating patterns an ongoing and regular part of your lifestyle. Therefore, I urge you to consider carefully the points already made in this chapter and to begin to put these strategies into practice. As pointed out above, too often dieters think of *how* they eat as window dressing to *what* they eat. That is not true. Part of long-term weight management is changing not only your eating patterns but how you *feel* about food and your relationship to it. That is why pleasure can be the make-or-break aspect of long-term weight loss and weight management success.

It goes without saying that a large part of the pleasure of eating a meal is the result of the look of the food, its aroma, consistency, temperature, and so on. As pointed out above, every food marketing and advertising executive knows that. Coffee smells robust and rich. Ice cream looks creamy and is deliciously cold on your tongue. No one can deny that what makes food pleasurable is not how many or what kind of vitamins or minerals it contains, but how it stimulates as many senses as possible.

But dieters deny themselves sensory pleasure, which is why most diets are short term and, ultimately, unsuccessful. As this chapter has been repeatedly stressing: Healthy eating is about *perceptions* and *expectations*. Losing weight is supposed to be boring and difficult, right? Diet foods are not supposed to taste good, right? The fact is that your *perception* of your goal ("I am going to suffer through another diet" versus "I am eating healthy and tasteful foods in a more responsible way") has *everything* to do with how reaching that goal *feels*.

To begin reeducating yourself that food is a source of pleasure rather than a source of pain, you must not only appreciate the food itself, but you must reevaluate your unstated assumptions about what makes food and eating "satisfying." To successfully incorporate all the other strategies into your life—strategies that can go a long way toward successful weight-loss and weight-management progress—you have to look at your personal assumptions about "satisfaction." In other words, you have to examine what "truths" you hold about gaining pleasure from food. As you worked through the first three levels of the pleasure pyramid, many of these assumptions may have already come to light.

I mentioned a common assumption that dieters hold: Dieting has to be painful and the food bland. If you hold that belief, then you can slow down and appreciate a beautifully prepared plate until the moon turns blue, but you will never feel that the asparagus and skinless chicken breast on your plate is truly satisfying. Your mind-set will interfere with your sensory pleasure. So it is time now for you to tackle the last step of the pleasure pyramid: bringing to consciousness unstated assumptions and personal beliefs about food and pleasure.

A stumbling block for many dieters is the belief that enjoying food means feeling full. As John Ash points out in the Foreword, it takes twenty minutes for you to realize your hunger is fully satisfied. If you eat quickly until you feel full, chances are that a little while later you will feel uncomfortably full. When you eat just to a feeling of satisfaction, you will have the pleasure of feeling comfortable in the hours after your meal, as well as during it.

The assumptions and beliefs that can detract from pleasure take many forms. Perhaps you have a pattern of sitting down to dinner and reviewing your day. If you are like many people, mealtime is the time to think back over the challenges and petty irritants of the day, strategizing how you can change things or how you might have done something differently. Such, mostly negative, "mind talk" is not conducive to appreciating a meal and feeling satisfied with what you ate.

Another way we deny ourselves pleasure is to believe that what was true long ago remains true today. If you have not tasted asparagus since you were six years old—a time when you probably rejected this and most other vegetables—then how do you know you still do not like it? No matter how much sensory pleasure you get from admiring the gorgeous diamond-patterned tips of the long, green, graceful asparagus stalks, you will reject the food as one you "don't like." But our tastes change as we grow up. Can you give up the decades-old assumption that you "hate asparagus" and give it another try?

The final strategy in this chapter is to, take the time now to examine your unstated assumptions and beliefs about your dining habits and food preferences. Explore how these current patterns and preferences could detract from increasing your enjoyment of eating healthfully and consciously.

Inner and Outer Satisfaction Exercise

Spend a half hour or so reviewing your food choices and eating history to see if you can identify assumptions, prejudices, and beliefs that have affected the satisfaction you get from eating. Then come up with strategies to test these assumptions to see if they are really true for you, or if they need testing and changing.

For example, do you always avoid certain foods, perhaps those you tried once and did not like or those you deem "health foods"? Why do you dislike these foods? Ask yourself a series of questions probing your assumptions about a particular food. How long has it been since you tried it? Can you allow for the possibility that you might like it now? Can you allow for the possibility that if it had been prepared in a different way you might find it satisfying? Perhaps you don't like broccoli by itself, but have you tried it as part of a stir-fry, where its taste blends with other vegetables? Maybe the broccoli you so disliked was overcooked and soggy. Perhaps you would like it raw and dipped in a fat-free sauce. Have you ever tried it that way? Perhaps you don't like broccoli because when you were a kid your father made you sit at the table until you ate it all, and so your dislike of this food really has nothing to do with the food but has to do with your resentment toward your father.

There are all kinds of hidden reasons we gravitate toward certain foods and avoid others. Our pleasure with eating and our food choices are often based on emotions rather than reason. So, while increasing the sensory pleasure of your dining experience improves your odds for long-term weight loss and management, also remember that your assumptions about what brings you pleasure are part of the equation.

Your basic self is the self that often forms the most deeply held assumptions and beliefs that make up your emotional approach to food. So, it is wise to spend as long as you need on this tier of the pleasure pyramid exploring these assumptions, testing them, and then devising strategies that bring the basic self into harmonious alliance with the conscious self.

In the past four chapters, we have focused on increasing awareness of your own needs and preferences. In Chapter 5 we are going to look at how interpersonal relationships can affect your weight management. Friends, family, and coworkers can either sabotage or help you in your efforts. Let us now see how you can enjoy being with others while staying on track with your own goals.

Chapter 5
Relationships: How Family and Friends Can Support or Sabotage Us

"After a good dinner, one can forgive anybody, even one's own relatives."

—Oscar Wilde

From the beginning of life, when we took nourishment from our mothers, food has been intertwined with our relationships. As a child, we may have bonded with our family members, sitting around the dinner table, talking about the day's events, sharing feelings, and forming values. As we moved into our adult years, food and wine may have become an integral part of our social relationships and even of our intimate ones. For anniversaries and other special occasions, we go out to eat at a restaurant. Holidays draw families and friends together, with everyone preparing their favorite dishes. Certainly sharing culinary delights can be one of life's greatest joys.

Unfortunately, relationships also often cause negative feelings that can contribute to emotional overeating. Your experiences at the family dinner table might have been more stressful than convivial. Your spouse or partner may be urging you to lose weight while bringing home cookies and other temptations from every shopping trip. Your friend may encourage you to go ahead "just this once" and have a second helping. Your mother or brother may refuse to serve anything that you can eat on your diet when you visit their home. "Don't be so difficult. We can't all change for you!" they may complain.

What is going on? Don't those who love and care about you want you to be healthy and happy? Yes, on a conscious level they do. But on an unconscious level, they may be waging their own battles, such as reacting to their own fear of change—either that you will change, or that they will be forced to change.

Since most of our relationships take place at least sometimes within the context of eating and drinking, any dietary change you make threatens the status quo. You are upsetting a comfortable, established pattern: the doughnut and coffee break with your coworker, the evening bowl of ice cream with your wife or husband, the popcorn at the movies with your child, the Friday afternoon drinks with your friends. Not only are you breaking a pattern in these relationships, but you may be reminding others of the need to take control of their own unhealthy habits. So, do not be surprised at the resistance and downright anger you may encounter from others as you make healthier choices in your own life. But also do not yield to these external pressures.

The information in this chapter will help you stay on course with your choice to lose weight and to maintain a lifestyle that will help you keep the weight off. The California Wine Country Diet relationship pyramid will take you step-by-step through some of the challenges you might face and suggest solutions and strategies for meeting these challenges.

The First Tier of the Relationship Pyramid: Relationship with Yourself

At the base of the relationship pyramid is the most important relationship of all—your relationship with yourself. This tier lays the foundation for all the others, because this step asks you to examine how you see the world and yourself in that world. So, before you prepare strategies for dealing with pressures from others, you would do well to explore how the greatest resistance you may have to deal with when making changes could come from yourself.

Take a few minutes to go back to tier 1 in Chapter 3, which deals with practicality. It was there that we talked about the conflicts that can arise between the emotional basic self and the rational conscious self. The basic self is the seat of our habitual behaviors, to which our basic self clings tenaciously. Consider your cherished habits: that latté you look forward to every morning, the rich and creamy cinnamon roll you treat yourself to at break, the salty chips you love to wash down with a cold beer while watching a game. Each of us has our favorite foods and beverages. When we prepare to "go on a diet," our basic self cringes at the thought of giving up these pleasurable habits. But we do so anyway—allowing our conscious self to take over in the name of losing weight. Then what happens when we successfully lose the weight? We go off the diet. We stop being conscious decision makers. Our basic self brokers for power—and usually gets it. We start slipping back into old habits, and we start regaining the weight we just worked so hard to lose. Why? Because we have not learned how to negotiate the tricky waters between the desires of our basic self and the wisdom of our conscious self.

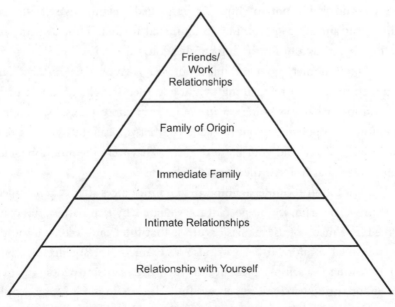

The Relationship Pyramid

By reviewing the material in Chapter 3 and your answers to the questions there, you will have a good sense of how much resistance you can expect to feel as you follow the California Wine Country Diet program. Although you are provided meal plans in Part II, which will make it easier for you to stay on course and provide "conscious indulgence" calories to satisfy your basic self, you can expect that your basic self will still continue to resist the good intentions of your conscious self. That is why it is so important for you to take seriously the additional work of gaining insight into yourself that you will be asked to undertake in this chapter.

In my clinical work as a psychotherapist working with people experiencing weight issues, I find that I spend most of my time dealing with my clients' feelings about themselves—particularly with their struggle to understand the *original sources* of their eating patterns and body images. For example, after some reflection, "Jan" was able to uncover the fact that she began to turn to food for comfort during junior high school, when her parents' divorce caused her intense inner pain and turmoil.

"David," however, realized that his weight problems started when he was laid off from a job he loved. He filled his empty hours with watching TV and eating potato chips. As he gained weight, his self-esteem, which was already compromised, plummeted further. This, in turn, affected his enthusiasm for finding another job.

Take a moment now to think about your own personal history. Can you identify a pattern of gaining weight and then struggling to lose it? If so, consider what was going on in your life at those times. Is there an emotional component to your food choices that you can uncover or probe for insight? Where did your pattern start? What were the emotional circumstances that fostered the original behavior?

In addition to understanding the circumstances that originally led to your weight gain, it is important to evaluate why that pattern has continued. For many of us, the basic truth is that food can become a source of emotional comfort. It helps us push away uncomfortable feelings. After all, eating is a sensory pleasure, so when the events or people in your life are upsetting you, you can always find pleasure in food. Many people have described food to me as "a friend who is always there." You do not have to dress up to eat. You do not have to be in a good mood to indulge your palate. Your favorite snack will never talk back, criticize, or reject you. Having a relationship with food takes a lot less effort than maintaining relationships with family, friends, and others.

In addition, weight can be a great excuse for avoiding fearful situations such as looking for a job or engaging in a romantic relationship. For many people, keeping weight on helps to maintain their fantasy of a better life to come. The logic goes something like this: "When I lose this weight, I'll be happy (or I'll get a promotion or I'll feel good about myself)." What is really going on here is that happiness (however it is defined) is deferred, because the person really has no intention of making the commitment to losing weight. So they use weight as an explanation for their not having what they really want. The weight becomes a screen keeping them from examining their real feelings, which may be that they do not believe they deserve to be happy, or promoted, or attain whatever their fantasy "perfect life" includes.

While there certainly is weight prejudice in our society, and people do tend to feel better when they lose weight, you are setting yourself up for dangerous disappointment and the regaining of any lost weight if you hold an expectation that by losing weight you will gain a perfect life. Life will go on pretty much the same way as it did before—only you will weigh less!

I am not trying to be cynical. The reality is that you may indeed find a new job or start a new romantic relationship once you lose weight and feel better about your physical self. However, sooner or later you will have to face the emotional patterns that led to your original weight problem, and you will also have to deal with the ever present stresses of daily living.

So I repeat: It is important to understand the underlying issues that have contributed to your weight gain and to reasons you have not succeeded in dealing with these issues. In this chapter, I can only raise the issue and ask you to spend some time reviewing your emotional history, not lead you through the process of deep self-exploration. Depending on your situation, you may want to work with a psychotherapist to gain depth of clarity on what you discover, or you may want to read the books listed in the "Suggested Reading and Resources" section at the back of this book. But whatever you do, please do not wait until you have lost weight to begin appreciating yourself. Start *today*.

Let me illustrate the important point I just made with the story of one of my clients who came to me for help with her binge-eating patterns. "Iris" works full time as a nurse at a large hospital and has two school-age children. She keeps a perfect house and describes her marriage as fairly happy, although she wishes her husband would help out more.

As we explored underlying issues, we focused on her family of origin, or the family in which she was raised. Iris described her mother as a traditional housewife who was always taking care of everyone else. Iris never remembers seeing her sitting down, unless it was to do something useful such as sewing or folding laundry. Iris was brought up with the values of not being selfish and of nurturing others and carried these values over into her relationship with her husband and kids.

As for her current eating patterns, Iris described them as "healthy and controlled" during the day. Her binge eating usually occurred later, after her family had gone to bed. While hating the feeling of being so out of control, Iris recognized that this binge eating was the one way she gave something to herself.

As we began working with the California Wine Country Diet principles in the Wheel of Weight-Management, Iris had no problems with the first three. She probably could have taught a course on nutrition, physical activity, and practicality. It was the principle of pleasure that she struggled with—the idea of slowing down and giving herself the pleasure of truly tasting the food she ate was entirely "too selfish." I asked her to begin shifting that pattern and belief by giving herself, at first, just one single minute to truly taste and enjoy the food she put in her mouth without doing anything else. In other words, she was to eat when she was eating, not eat while she did several other chores.

She followed this advice, and over time she gradually increased her "mindful" eating time until she was able to give herself a full half hour every day after work to sit down, relax, have a cup of tea or glass of wine and a bite to eat, and just be with herself. As a result of this one simple behavior change, Iris was amazed at the increase in her energy level. Having a healthier relationship with herself actually increased her energy so that she could devote herself even more attentively to others, which was something she valued and needed in her life. She stopped her pattern of binge eating and now proudly proclaims that she enjoys the pleasure of her own company.

It is important that you seek out the underlying patterns, beliefs, and behaviors of your perceived eating problems or weight-loss and weight-management challenges. The more seriously you take this inner foundational work, the better your chances of long-term success in your shift toward healthy living. Work through the sections below to begin probing into these often unconscious patterns.

Affirming What You Want

How is your relationship with yourself? Do you enjoy your own company? While some of us need more alone time than others, it is important for each of us to have time to recharge our batteries, step back from life, and get reacquainted with ourselves. There are times, such as when you have a baby to care for, that alone time is very hard to come by. Often, however, the problem is that we simply do not *allow* ourselves quality time alone.

In our society, "doing" is highly valued. Relaxing by yourself is considered "doing nothing." We are supposed to be active, involved, and productive. But, of course, we must find balance in all things, which includes getting to know ourselves and spending time alone relaxing.

So, think about what you would like to do by yourself on a daily basis. How could time with yourself enhance your implementing the California Wine Country Diet program? The best way for you to truly appreciate the new foods (and wine, if you drink alcohol) that you will be trying out is by yourself. How about giving yourself time each day for at least one experience in which you eat by yourself and relish each morsel? What other activities would you like to do alone that have nothing to do with food and wine? Reading? Taking a bath? Taking a walk? Begin to make time for them.

Enjoying Your Relationship with Yourself

Once you have made time for yourself, the next step is finding ways to appreciate who you are. Do you treat yourself well? For instance, do you take the same care when preparing a meal for yourself that you would if you were preparing it for a guest? If not, why not? Why not use the best dishes and finest silverware for yourself? Why not light some candles and put on some mood music even if you are eating alone? Begin to do some things related to food and eating that show you value yourself.

Or, at the other end of the spectrum, cut loose and have fun. If you tend to be strict or overly serious with yourself, cut loose and shake up your ingrained patterns. Eat dessert first. Eat with your hands. Go ahead and lick the bowl! Listen to that child inside you and let him or her out to play. No one is watching, and we all need a break from the responsibilities of adulthood. We need to tap into our true likes and dislikes. It is amazing what a difference spending a half hour doing what *you* want to do and shaking up old, ingrained, and unconscious patterns can make in your life.

The Second Tier of the Relationship Pyramid: Intimate Relationships

Remember when you first fell in love? You probably lost your appetite. It is a common side effect of the rush of emotion. In fact, many aspects of our intimate relationships have a bearing on our physiology, including our eating patterns and food choices. On the positive side is the enjoyment of sharing food and wine with a loved one. The sensuality of one enhances the sensuality of the other. Certain foods such as chocolate and oysters are said to have aphrodisiac qualities. We express our love by preparing a special meal or taking our loved one to a particular restaurant.

On the other hand, relationships can affect our eating habits in negative ways. When a relationship sours or is seriously stressed, we tend to alleviate our sorrows or comfort ourselves through food. But even happy events can have potentially negative effects. For example, when people marry, they tend to begin to gain weight over time. Richard Stuart and Barbara Jacobson explore this phenomenon in their book *Weight, Sex and*

Marriage. In their survey of 15,000 respondents, they found that happily married women gained an average of 18.4 pounds in the first thirteen years of marriage, while those in unhappy marriages gained 42.6 pounds. Husbands in happy marriages gained 19 pounds and in unhappy marriages gained an average of 38 pounds. What is going on?

The authors found that those who are happy in their marriages tend to follow a pattern of gradual weight gain because marriage or long-term partnership is often seen as a license to relax.[1] We now have the security of our partner's acceptance and we are out of the competitive single world. Plus, when you are happy, your weight is less likely to impact your sense of self-worth, so you have less motivation to change. What is more, married couples often take on a more sedentary lifestyle: one of their primary forms of recreation is to cook at home or eat out at a restaurant. For women, there is the added component of pregnancy.

The weight-gain pattern in unhappy marriages is far more complex. Food can serve both men and women as a substitute for affection and lack of sexual intimacy. Food can ease emotional pain, and, unlike your spouse, you can count on it to always be there. Using food this way may become addictive and can result in significant weight gain. While we might feel physically hungry a few times a day, emotional hunger can be with us continually.

In addition to the role eating plays in a marriage, Stuart and Jacobson examined the role weight can play in a marriage relationship. While the number-one reason people give for losing weight is to be attractive to the opposite sex, keeping weight on serves many purposes. Eating can be a way to stuff down anger, and weight can be an act of rebellion against the person who is trying to get you to lose weight. Weight can serve as a protection from unwanted sexual intimacy or feared sexual feelings. Weight can help keep a marriage together by warding off infidelity. Spouses may feel threatened when their partner loses weight and begins getting more attention from others. Weight loss can upset the power balance within a relationship.[2]

I report all this information to urge you to pay attention to the state of your intimate relationships as you begin the California Wine Country Diet program. Examine what has happened in the past when you lost weight and tried to keep it off. Was your partner supportive then? Is he or she now? Are there subtle ways he or she sabotages your efforts? Does your partner also need to lose weight? If so, does he or she want to join you on the diet program?

Affirming What You Want

Ideally, you have a partner who truly supports you and is happy to eat according to the California Wine Country Diet principles. If this is the case, you can begin a new adventure together that will enhance both your health and relationship. Sit down and go over the program together. Who is going to be responsible for planning, buying, and preparing the food? How are you going to account for different calorie levels and food preferences? What kind of support do you want from each other? Is it all right for your partner to comment when you are not following the plan?

What do you do if you are with a partner who does not support you in your endeavor to lose weight? The reasons for nonsupport are varied. If it stems from your partner's insecurity, you can try to reassure him or her that you are going on the diet for your health and because you care about yourself and him or her. In some cases, over time, your partner may be persuaded to make healthier choices for himself or herself. On the other hand, the best approach may be to just start the program without any announcements. Once you are feeling confident in your commitment, talk to your partner about what you are doing, share your feelings, and encourage your partner to share his or her feelings.

Whatever is going on in your intimate relationship, it is essential to remember that the most important relationship you have is the one with yourself. To be successful you cannot allow your food selections to be controlled by your partner's moods and choices. As you will see when we talk about the other relationships in your life, setting boundaries is essential.

Enjoying Food and Wine
in an Intimate Relationship

The joys of sharing food and wine with someone you love are immense. They can range from cooking dinner together with romantic music playing, to sharing a cup of tea in front of a crackling fire, to sipping a glass of your favorite wine on the deck, to licking whipped cream off your partner's body. The California Wine Country Diet program encourages you to make food and wine part of your loving relationship. Bringing pleasure and variety into your culinary experiences together will enhance your delight in food and wine and enrich your relationship. Take a moment now to brainstorm some ideas for making healthy food choices a positive experience in your relationship.

The Third Tier of the Relationship Pyramid: Your Immediate Family

With your own immediate family, especially your children, you have the opportunity to set new patterns related to food that are healthy and that strengthen your relationships. Researchers who study childhood obesity have found that the decline in the number of families who sit down together to eat meals has been a significant contributor to childhood weight gain. "Absence of family meals is associated with lower fruit and vegetable consumption as well as consumption of more fried food and carbonated beverages."[3] At the family dinner table, you have the chance to prepare healthy meals, watch what your children eat, and converse. It is important to make this a positive time rather than a time to grill your children about their homework or admonish them about misbehavior. Try to keep the emotional associations of eating and family in the realm of the positive and nurturing.

If you have not been having family dinners, you might want to introduce them slowly into your family's routine, perhaps one or two nights a week to start. Then keep them going.

While the food plans and recipes in the California Wine Country Diet are designed for adults, they can be adapted easily for children and teenagers. Be sure to review the recommendations for children in the *Dietary Guidelines for Americans 2005*. You can download these at www.healthierus.gov/dietaryguidelines. Some of the dishes you will be incorporating into your new culinary lifestyle may be unfamiliar to your children, so it might be best to introduce these into their diet slowly, while continuing to serve them some of their old favorites.

Take some time now to think about your family and the nutritional and emotional needs of your children. Depending on their ages and temperaments, each child may require that you approach him or her using a different strategy, especially if you are attempting to dramatically change your family's nutritional and physical activity pattern. You are up against the forces of commerce, which endlessly promote high fat and high sugar foods to children. You are also confronting children's drastically reduced levels of physical activity. Television, computers, video games, and other technological entertainment have kept children sedentary. You will not be able to change their habits overnight, or even very easily. Fortunately, with the recent media attention on the dangers of childhood obesity, you will find support in the larger community. Exciting things are happening in the schools including school vegetable gardens and bans on sodas and vending machine snacks. Find out what your child's school is doing in this area.

There are also subtle educational actions you can take at home. For example, you could rent the movie *Supersize Me* and watch it with your children to educate them about the consequences of eating too much fast food or not paying attention to portion size. The key is to subtly work in ideas that can help change your children's attitudes, as you also gradually encourage better food choices and increased physical activity. Be creative when it comes to mentoring them into new ways of thinking and being. For example, you could enlist the help of your children in planting a garden, however small. Fruits and vegetables will even grow in containers on a deck or porch. Most kids are delighted when they see the efforts of their labors, and they are usually eager to eat the fruits and vegetables they have grown themselves. They not only learn valuable skills, increase their activity level, and eat fresh foods, but they can have a lot of fun, too. With a little imagination, improving your relationship with your children can be an integral part of your success on the California Wine Country Diet.

Affirming What You Want

Imagine a typical day at your house as you would like it to be. What are your children eating for breakfast, lunch, and dinner? How are they getting the physical activity they need? How can dinner be a time that supports and promotes family closeness? What activities could you do where everyone would be entertained? Brainstorm ideas and then put one or two into action right away. Gradually institute other changes, and ask your children and spouse for their ideas and input as well, so that everyone in the family is involved.

Enjoying Your Immediate Family Relationships

It is so easy to get caught up in the demands of making a living, driving kids to sports and after-school activities, and overseeing their homework that we often lose sight of what is most important for our children. As we have discussed, taking care of their health through sound nutrition and encouraging physical activity are two of the most important responsibilities of parenthood. But you cannot legislate change for your family. They will likely only rebel at being told that something is "good" for them. Instead, incorporate healthy food choices and physical activity into moments of family fun. Allow children to learn and grow and change, not by "educating" them, but instead by simply pursuing enjoyable activities that subtly teach lessons.

We have already talked about some creative ideas you could try. But push the envelope and come up with more ideas that will make healthy food a positive aspect of your family relationships. For example, if you involve your children in food preparation, they will tend to see it not as a chore but as a fun activity you can do together. It will also help build their foundation for selecting healthy foods and develop their sense of competency. You could plan a berry-picking day. Carve a pumpkin, and then go on the Internet and find a pumpkin recipe to make together. Visit a local farm or farmers' market and actually talk to the people who grow or harvest the food. Allow your child to pick an unusual fruit or vegetable from the store on every shopping trip. Research the country where it came from, and allow the child to cut the unusual fruit or vegetable into portions so that every family member can try it—and rate it. All these activities help children to feel closer to the world of nature, deepen their appreciation for the food they eat, enhance their desire to try new foods, and spend quality time in a family activity. You will be helping your children and yourself at the same time.

Fourth Tier of the Relationship Pyramid: Your Family of Origin

As an adult, getting together with your family of origin (the one you grew up in) can cause you to quickly slip back into childhood preferences, feelings, and emotional patterns—even if you no longer identify with those preferences, feelings, or patterns. One of my clients, "Dan," has a story that is quite revealing in this regard. He told me how every time he went to visit his mother she would fix a macaroni and cheese dish that had been his favorite as a boy. He would exclaim his delight and appreciation even though he had stopped liking this dish long before he graduated from high school. One evening as his mother piled on a third serving, he finally found the courage to tell her that he did not want any more. His mother replied, "But you've always loved my macaroni and cheese!"

"Mom, it's you I've always loved. I stopped liking macaroni and cheese about twenty years ago."

"Oh, my dear," his mother exclaimed, finally admitting her own feelings. "I can't stand the stuff myself! I just made it because I thought you wanted it and expected it."

They both had a hearty laugh. The next night Dan took his mother out to dinner to enjoy the start of his new, more adult and truthful relationship with her.

Traditional foods can be a treasured tie to the past, but they can also be an anchor that pulls you away from your commitment to a healthier lifestyle. Before you spend time with your family of origin, prepare yourself. If their eating patterns are generally similar to those of the California Wine Country Diet, then you face few challenges. Your most difficult choice will be to resist large portion sizes and second helpings.

If your family eats foods that are very different from the California Wine Country Diet, your best approach is to bring a dish that fits with the diet as a contribution to the meal. If you are with your family for a longer visit, offer to help with food shopping and preparation. How much you want to say about your diet is an individual choice. You may want to wait until you are well on your way in the program before bringing it up, because once you have experienced success, it is a lot easier to discuss what you are doing with others. Diets are such a major topic of interest in this country that when you mention you are on one, you are bound to elicit more opinions and advice than you care to hear. Everyone wants to offer opinions about what diet works best, what foods you should eat or avoid, and the like. Sometimes keeping a low profile is a lot easier than engaging in such debates.

But you might be quite surprised by your family, as I was on a recent visit to my eighty-nine-year-old stepmother, Audrey Logan, who lives in an assisted-living facility. Arriving exhausted and famished after the long drive, I was not at all sure what I would find to eat, for she takes almost all her meals in the community dining room, and I knew that because of the late hour the kitchen would be closed. What is more, she is confined to a wheelchair and on twenty-four-hour-a-day oxygen, so her ability to prepare a meal is seriously limited. Nevertheless, suspecting that I would be hungry, she had prepared some food for me. I was delighted to be served sliced heirloom tomatoes, which had been handpicked from the communal garden. They were topped with an olive tapenade she had purchased at the local co-op. Also on the plate were slices of organic Vermont cheddar cheese and Ak-mak whole wheat crackers. To top it off, she served me a chilled individual-sized bottle of California Chardonnay, which she keeps for special occasions. I had been so excited to tell her about my new book, and here she was presenting me with a perfect California Wine Country Diet meal!

I could not help chuckling, for my stepmother and I had spent years quibbling about food. Her cooking style had been basic American—meat and potatoes—and she could never remember which food fad I was following when I came home to visit. Was I eating meat or not? Was I swearing off wheat? Was I eating only low-fat foods? Now here we were, decades later, enjoying exactly the same kinds of foods. When anyone says that the California Wine Country Diet is too much work, I think about her and the fabulous meal we shared, which was doubly enriched—we not only shared delicious and healthy food, but we shared a loving relationship.

Here in the United States, we are starting to accept much of the nutritional wisdom of our parents and grandparents, common sense that was derailed by the explosion of "manufactured" food in the 1950s.

One of the best pieces of advice I came across recently was a suggestion to go back to the older cookbooks because the portions are smaller. When you visit your family, especially your elders, inquire into their early eating habits and food experiences. Their stories can be delightful as well as instructive.

Affirming What You Want

Before your next visit to your family of origin, spend some time thinking about what you want the experience to be like. While you cannot undo the past, you can change how you respond in the present. How will you stay true to the principles of the California Wine Country Diet during your visit? What is important for your relationship with family members at this time? If you have always gone along with what others dictate, maybe it is time to stand up for what you are now doing. If you have spent your visits in the past trying to persuade your family to adopt your point of view, maybe it is time to focus on listening to them. Imagine what a positive visit would look like. See your family having a good time together, and see yourself staying centered on your own plan.

Enjoying Your Family of Origin Relationships

Another important strategy in your relationships is to expand what you bring to them. If you are going to visit your family, why *not* take a dish to share? That way you will be making a thoughtful gesture while also ensuring that you will have at least one food choice that fits with your plan.

Parents and siblings usually feel that they do not get to spend enough time together. So why not spend some quality one-on-one time with a family member by suggesting a walk together? Even in the most couch-potato prone family, there's usually someone who would rather get out in the fresh air before or after dinner. Or, suggest a game that was a family favorite or a new one that will bring everyone together and away from the television set. With a little imagination and sincere attention, you can create moments for your family that will not only serve your needs but help bring the family closer together.

The Top of the Relationship Pyramid:
Friends and Work Relationships

Relationships with friends and coworkers present some of the same challenges you encounter in dealing with your own family and your extended family: You are bound to find yourself in eating situations with people who may or may not share your dietary beliefs and preferences. You may feel torn between the needs of the relationship and your own needs. Your temptations may come in many guises. You might find yourself feeling like "Susan," whom you met in Chapter 3. When she gathered with friends, her basic self rebelled against her conscious self's decision to limit portion size, protesting inwardly, "I should be able to eat whatever they eat!"

Or you may identify more closely with "Mary," another of my clients. The highlight of her day was going to lunch with the coworkers she had grown close to over their fifteen years of working together. But as she gained more and more weight, she feared that her only choice might be to give up these treasured lunches and bring her lunch from home.

Or perhaps "Peter's" situation more closely matches your own. Peter was doing well losing weight until it came time for a party or business event, which, unfortunately, was a routine part of his work life. Caught up in the whirl of business socializing, he soon lost track of how much wine he had drunk and found it impossible to control his food choices.

Your situation may be different, but generally speaking, social situations present some of our toughest challenges. We lose our focus and resolve in social situations for a variety of reasons, but mostly because our emotional basic self takes over. Think back to your own childhood and how you got swayed to do things by peer pressure or found it difficult to stand up for your own choices or preferences. When it comes to eating and drinking patterns, we are often torn between not wanting to stand out and not wanting to be left out. It is so much easier to just go along with the crowd. Everyone else is indulging (or overindulging) and, besides, that cake looks *so* good. Your basic self is likely to begin its bargaining—or badgering: "It's just not fair that I have to be on this diet when they're eating everything they want! If I don't eat the cake everyone will know that I'm on a diet." And so goes the inner, often unconscious battle, between our basic and conscious selves.

Once again, the key is to return to your relationship with yourself. Think about what is really important to you in the social situation and what your alternatives might be. With close friends, just as with family members, try first asking for the support you need.

Mary, for example, decided to ask her friends to go to another restaurant for lunch, where she could select healthier choices and be less tempted by the rich food of their usual restaurant. It turned out that they enjoyed the new restaurant, and everyone was actually grateful to Mary for suggesting it.

Sometimes, you might want to skip certain social functions all together, at least during your transition into the California Wine Country Diet program. At the very least, you need to do some advanced planning. For instance, Peter, who had to attend many social functions in the course of business, found he could turn down invitations without adversely affecting his business or social relationships. And he started a practice of mentally preparing himself for those he did attend. He made an agreement between his conscious and basic selves to limit his wine to two glasses and then to switch to nonalcoholic beverages. When someone tried to fill his glass with wine, he would say that he was the designated driver. When faced with a mouth-watering buffet, his strategy was to get a single plate of what he really wanted and then go off to eat it by himself. After enjoying this food, he focused on the social aspects of the evening. At sit-down dinners, he tried to consciously choose what he was going to eat at the beginning of each course.

Both Mary and Peter found a solution to their challenge by practicing a foundational principle of the California Wine Country Diet program: conscious indulgence. Even when you are at a business or social affair where the servings are small, in the thrall of the festivities you can quickly lose track of how much you are eating and drinking. By remembering to use your intellectual, rational self to set limits, you can find a way to satisfy the desires of your basic self *and* stay on course with your weight-loss or weight-management goals.

Affirming What You Want

Think about the social situations in your life. Are they meeting your relationship needs? How do they support your ability to follow the California Wine Country Diet? How do they sabotage your efforts? Now consider how you can increase your support from friends and coworkers. Brainstorm ways to set limits for your basic self while also allowing yourself the pleasures of your social and business relationships and experiences.

Enjoying Your Relationships with Friends and Coworkers

While we have been looking at ways that social situations can make it difficult to stay with a food plan, your social relationships are an integral part of your success. You may find yourself moving away from some friends because they are not as focused on healthy living as you are. You may be surprised, as Mary was, that you can introduce your friends to healthy California Wine Country Diet foods and that they will enjoy them.

Brainstorm ways to transform your present social patterns into patterns that are more supportive of you. For example, perhaps instead of always meeting friends at restaurants, where you have less control over your food choices, you could initiate a Supper Club, where you and your friends rotate hosting a get-together at your homes. If you tend to meet with friends and coworkers in situations that focus on food, then find ways to alter that focus away from eating. Go out dancing, meet for a game night, go out to a movie—just take the focus of the activity off of eating. There are many, many ways to have fun with your friends and to entertain business contacts that can enhance your pleasure while keeping you on track with your health and weight-loss goals. You just have to plan ahead a bit to put these ideas into action.

We have one final aspect of the Wheel of Weight-Management to consider: Variety. We met this aspect briefly in this chapter, but variety goes much deeper than finding ways to lessen food temptations while fostering relationships. It applies to your entire life. As you have learned previously, one of the major reasons for failing in your diet is that you grow bored with your food choices and with your exercise program. While we are creatures of habit, we also rebel against our habits. If we do not have variety in our diet and our activities, we tend to lose our good intentions before a new habit is well formed. So let us complete our journey around the Wheel of Weight-Management by exploring the important subject of variety.

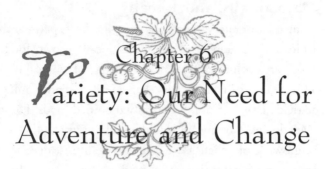

Chapter 6
Variety: Our Need for Adventure and Change

Variety's the very spice of life.
—*William Cowper*

The well-known saying that heads this chapter is a part of our collective folk wisdom. But how often have you said it without truly reflecting on its meaning? Despite sometimes getting us into trouble, our desire for variety motivates us to explore, and it makes life more exciting. Just as spices add flavor and interest to your food, sprinkling variety throughout your California Wine Country Diet will keep the program interesting and is a key to successfully turning it into a long-term lifestyle.

On the other hand, you may be thinking that too many choices and too much variety adds stress to your life. And who needs more stress? In fact, part of the reason we establish habits, such as choosing the same foods and the same label of wine over and over, is because we are happy with what we know. But the problem with not being curious enough to explore change and add variety to your life is that you stop paying attention; you do things by rote. As regards food, when you limit your nutritional variety, you also tend to disregard portion size as you unconsciously overeat familiar foods. In this chapter we will explore the value of increasing the variety in your life and diet. This last section of the Wheel of Weight Management is detailed in the California Wine Country Diet variety pyramid.

The First Tier of the Variety Pyramid:
Eating Seasonally and Locally

You can incorporate variety into your life by experimenting with seasonal fruits and vegetables and choosing locally grown foods. These kinds of foods are an integral part of the cuisine of the California wine country. This area of the country has taken a lead in championing chemical-free, pesticide-free, and non-genetically modified foods. For example, in 2003, Mendocino County became the first county in the country to outlaw the growing of genetically modified organisms, or GMOs. That the support for this ban came from a broad cross section of the community, including a majority of the grape growers and vineyard owners, indicates increasing concern over the safety of our food supply. It also demonstrates that citizens and small farmers can work together on a local level to stem the monopoly of impersonal multinational corporations that have taken over agriculture in the United States.

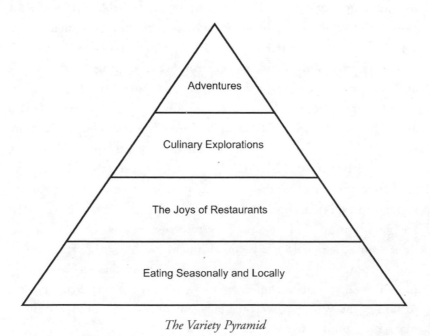

The Variety Pyramid

One taste of a home- or locally grown organic tomato is all it takes to convince most of us that what we get from the average grocery store is at best an imitation of what Mother Nature intended tomatoes to be. That is why so many grassroots groups and organized associations across the nation are raising their voices against genetically modified foods and the "big agribusiness" way of growing crops, which depends on using high dosages of pesticides and chemical fertilizers and harvesting foods before they are at peak ripeness and flavor.

By choosing locally grown vegetables and fruits as they come into season, and also by choosing organic foods when possible, you not only get to enjoy great-tasting food while improving your health, but you also add your voice to thousands of others who are making the statement that what we put in our bodies matters.

No matter what your opinion about the need to keep our food supply as pure as possible, you would be doing yourself a delightful favor by exploring your local sources of fresh produce and other foods. If you have never visited your local farmers' market—and most communities, even metropolitan ones, have at least one—then you are missing out on great fun and a satisfying culinary experience. Most of the foods you will find there will have been grown by small farmers in your immediate area or state, so the vegetables and fruits are fresh, some picked the same day they go on sale. Plus, many markets offer other wares such as delectable baked goods, fresh dairy products, and homemade jams. Many are organic and are made with pride by families who have had a relationship with the earth for generations.

While some foods at farmers' markets can be priced slightly higher than grocery store versions, they more than make up for the cost in their freshness, healthfulness, and taste. What is truly gratifying about becoming a regular at a farmers' market or food co-op is the relationships you can form with the local growers who sell their stock there. Most are happy to talk about their produce and other stock, and their stories are usually engaging. Then when you go home and make that delicious and healthy stir-fry, it is like inviting the farmers into your kitchen. No more anonymous heads of lettuce. Instead, your food will have a name and face to it: the red leaf lettuce from Joe and Jan's farm, the apples from the Prestons' place, and the organic cheese from Sam's goat herd.

Alice Waters, who has been called the "mother of modern American cooking" and owns the world-famous Chez Panisse restaurant in Berkeley, California, says of farmers' markets: "Yes, it takes a little longer to shop at the farmers' market, but what you get, in my mind, is an experience that enriches one's life. It's an experience of connecting with people. It smells good. It tastes good. It has a good feeling about it. There's no way that that kind of experience can't seduce people and make the supermarket experience in comparison pretty depressing."[1]

You might also like to investigate heirloom plants. These are open-pollinated varieties of plants. Unlike plants grown from hybrid seeds, the seeds from heirloom plants can be saved and planted to produce the same variety of food year after year.

For more information on farmers' markets and eating seasonally, visit www.seasonalchef.com. To find farmers' markets in various areas of the United States go to the Agricultural Marketing Service of the United States Department of Agriculture at www.ams.usda.gov. To learn more about preserving open-pollinated heirloom vegetables, fruits, and nuts, you can go to www.seedsavers.org.

If you plant and grow your own fruits and vegetables, eating locally and seasonally is already an integral part of your life. Adding variety for you may mean branching out into new varietals or new produce choices. For those readers who do not garden, now may be the time to give it a try.

Start small, perhaps with container tomatoes or a small herb plot. Once you have the satisfaction of tasting a soup you flavored with fresh, homegrown vegetables and herbs, I suspect you will be hooked and will plan a more ambitious garden the next year. Gardening also is a great way to get the whole family involved in paying more attention to food and diet and to healthy choices. And it is good exercise.

Eating Seasonally and Locally Exercise

Choose from the following options, or come up with your own ideas and begin to add variety to your culinary life.

- Check out the Web sites listed in this section to learn more about farmers' markets.

- Research the foods and wines produced in your local area or state, and what is available season to season.
- Brainstorm new ideas for how you could enjoy eating this locally grown produce in new ways.
- Pick out what you might want to grow and explore the option of organic gardening, container gardening, or gardening with heirloom seeds.

The Second Tier of the Variety Pyramid: The Joys of Restaurants

There is no easier path to culinary variety than eating in a restaurant. It used to be that you had to live in a metropolitan area to experience unusual cuisine, such as Thai, Caribbean, or Vietnamese. But today, in cities and towns large and small, there is an abundance of dining choices. In this case, to add variety to your culinary life all it takes is the curiosity to try something new. In addition to providing you the experience of new and different kinds of foods, restaurants also reduce your stress—someone else is doing the cooking and the dishes—and enliven your social life. If you are lucky, you might even get to indulge your senses with a view of the ocean or a nearby mountain.

No matter where you live and how numerous your restaurant choices, you probably tend to frequent the same two or three restaurants, getting in a culinary rut by ordering the same few dishes. Now is the time to widen your food horizons. As you know, the California Wine County Diet program encourages you to experiment with new types of cuisine and to expand your palate by trying unfamiliar dishes; restaurants are a prime place to practice this.

Another way to expand your choices is to be inventive in your own kitchen. The restaurant recipes in *The California Wine Country Diet* can be an important contribution to your success at losing and maintaining weight, but they also are meant to prompt you to believe in yourself as a cook. While there is no doubt that you can lose weight simply by following the general food plans, why not challenge yourself to add some spice to your life by trying out one of the suggested restaurant recipes each week. The recipes come from chefs across the

California wine country and are likely to introduce you to new spices, ingredients, and ways of preparing food. They are all thoroughly tested for ease of preparation, nutritional composition, and taste. I have no doubt that you will love them.

An added benefit to preparing the restaurant recipes is that it will educate you in the preparation of restaurant food. Many of the recipes have had adjustments made to the ingredients to lower fat or calorie content. Most have been adjusted for portion size to fit in with the different calorie levels of the meal plan. I have included with each revised recipe the original restaurant ingredients and portion sizes so that you can easily compare what you would be getting at the restaurant if you ordered this dish and adjust your dining experience accordingly to stay on track with your weight-loss program.

In terms of weight management, eating at restaurants can be problematic because the same plate of food comes to a 130-pound woman and to a 250-pound man. While in this book you will learn how to calculate your ideal calorie level and to judge correct portion sizes to meet this level, when you go to a restaurant you give part of that control over to the chef. It is up to you—through your motivation and willpower—to eat only what will keep you on track in your weight-loss program. Meat portions in restaurants, for example, are usually six to ten ounces, and sometimes far more. The recommended portion size for a petite woman would be about two or three ounces. So you can see that eating out can take some self-confidence and self-discipline. We will talk about ideas for measuring or judging portion size in Chapter 8.

In addition to the pitfalls of portion size in restaurant dining, it is difficult to know what is really in the food you are eating. The restaurant's job is to please customers so that they will come back. Fat, sugar, and salt all can make food more appealing and tasty. More healthful choices are dishes that leave these items out and are flavored with herbs and spices. This is the choice of most of the restaurants of the California wine country. With a little forethought, you can choose a restaurant that makes these healthful choices. And when in doubt about the content of a menu item, ask the chef how it is prepared. Most are happy to discuss this with you. It is also a wise idea to educate yourself about the terms used in cooking. For example, the following descriptive terms are good indicators for food that is prepared in a way that reduces fat content: steamed, broiled, roasted, poached, baked, grilled, and barbecued. With grilled and barbecued food, you have to make sure they were not cooked with a lot of butter or high-sugar sauces.

The Joys of Restaurants Exercise

Select one or more of the following options to put into practice in your life immediately:

- Make a list of the restaurants you have never visited, and try one or two.
- Review the Chapter 3 suggestions for restaurant eating, and write down those that you find most helpful. Put these strategies into play in your life.
- Look over the recipes of the restaurants in the California Wine Country Diet in Chapter 12. What can you learn from them about preparation and ingredients for when you go out to eat?
- Mark those recipes that you most want to try to cook at home yourself.

The Third Tier of the Variety Pyramid: Culinary Explorations

For some readers the foods mentioned in *The California Wine Country Diet* will be familiar. For others they may be foreign. For all of you, this will be an opportunity to try different foods that are nutritious and support your goal of weight loss. Some of the foods in the daily meal plans are those of the traditional Mediterranean diet, such as eggplant and olives. Some recipes use Asian sauces, some the spices of Latin American cuisine. Other foods are geared toward the American lifestyle, such as pizza. Keep an open mind and explore new items. You will probably find some foods that you never want to see again and others that will become keys to your long-term weight maintenance. You will never know until you try them.

As you are getting used to the food plans and restaurant recipes, you may feel that you have all the variety you can handle. Especially as you move into the "Forever After" part of the California Wine Country Diet, it will be important to continue experimentation. This can be as simple as selecting one food and trying a different variation of it each week. Instead of eating the same kind of bread every morning, go to a bakery and choose a novel flavored loaf. Or perhaps take a few moments the next time you are in a grocery store with an olive bar to sample a variety of olives. You might not have time in your life right now for gourmet cooking, but you could become an expert in seasonal fruits and vegetables. Exploration can be broad across categories or it can go deeply into one area.

Wine, of course, presents a world of endless of variety. Most wineries give wine tastings for free or at minimal cost. There are frequent wine tastings at other venues such as wine shops and festivals. Many of these are accompanied by food sampling. Increasingly, certain foods have become the center of attention themselves at festivals. In the California wine country, we have festivals devoted almost exclusively to tomatoes, garlic, mushrooms, crab, mustard, chocolate, olives, peaches, and apples. Each season brings the excitement of enjoying these foods at their freshest. Look for events in your area that will broaden your appreciation of local produce. For instance, in most areas you will find small local farmers who offer pick-your-own blueberries, apples, and other fruits. Have some fun by making an orchard visit a family affair, perhaps even packing a picnic lunch.

Culinary exploration can also take place from the most unlikely of places—your own couch or armchair. Your local Public Broadcasting station and the cable Food Network feature premier chefs, who provide instruction on preparing everything from roasts to crème bruleé. Then there are the multitude of cookbooks, magazines, and cooking Web sites to peruse. At the back of this book, you will find a listing of such resources. If you decide to move beyond your armchair, you may want to take a community cooking class. This can be a delightful way to meet new people and to increase your cooking skills.

No matter how you add variety to your life, above all do not let anything stop your culinary exploration. Let each season open a new door of discovery. If you like to cook, there are endless opportunities to increase your repertoire. If cooking is not for you, focus on finding new foods and expanding your appreciation. When you are paying close attention to what you are tasting, you are much less likely to fall into the greatest danger to your weight-loss program—overeating.

Culinary Explorations Exercise

Make a list of the foods and beverages you currently do not know much about or have never tried but would like to. Set yourself goals for exploring these choices. For example, set a goal that you will try one new vegetable a week or that you will explore California Chardonnays. Visit FoodTV.com and see which nutrition or cooking shows will be on and either watch them or record them for later viewing. Visit bookstores or libraries to look at cookbooks and magazines. Select a few that most appeal to you. On your first reading, view them like a travel log. Do not put any pressure on yourself to select recipes to try out. Enjoy the dishes vicariously. Perhaps after a while you may return to certain recipes and give them a try.

Top of the Variety Pyramid: Adventures

The word *adventure* refers to an undertaking that involves risk. Beyond this basic definition, adventure is a highly individual matter. For one person it may mean getting on a roller coaster, but for another the challenge may be a merry-go-round. When you are twenty, adventure might mean hitchhiking around Europe. When you are seventy, adventure may mean taking the Napa Valley Wine Train. Adventures entail not only undertaking activities that you find enjoyable but also pushing your boundaries a bit, trying new things or facing your preconceptions or fears.

Adventures will add variety to your life and your weight management program. I identify three levels of adventure: small, mid-sized, and large. Small adventures are those daily changes of routine that serve to make life a little more interesting—and, for our purposes, that add variety to your weight-loss program. A small adventure, then, might be eating out on your deck rather than in the den in front of the television. It might be growing a small pot of basil or trying out a new machine at the gym. Small adventures can be added to your life with minimal extra time or cost. They can turn a monotonous week into one that makes you appreciate your life a little more.

Mid-sized adventures are those that take slightly more planning and time, and begin to push a little on your comfort zone. If you have never exercised, adding a nightly walk is a mid-sized adventure. If you have never tried Thai food, choosing that kind of restaurant for your next night out might make you a bit anxious but can also add the thrill of discovery to your life. Mid-sized adventures invite novelty into your life as you explore choices that take you beyond the comfort zone of your normal routine.

Large adventures, as you can guess, are those that not only require a greater time, and perhaps financial, commitment but that also challenge you to discover new aspects of yourself. All of you reading this book may be at the beginning of a large adventure if you make a commitment to remake yourself, starting with losing weight through the California Wine Country Diet program. After all, this is not a diet program as much as it is a lifestyle change, a new way of appreciating yourself, honoring your health, and making wise food choices that you commit to for the long term.

You cannot remake your lifestyle without deep self-inquiry and self-discovery, and as you gain confidence and insight, you allow room for changes that could be classified as "large adventures."

Another large adventure might be redecorating your house to make your environment more pleasurable or just redoing your kitchen so it is more conducive to cooking. After you lose significant weight, you could make shopping for new clothes a large adventure by going to stores you never had the courage to visit before or trying out a completely new style. Perhaps you will even get a new hairstyle to go along with your new clothes.

If you have been self-conscious because of your weight, a large adventure for you might mean finally wearing a bathing suit or taking a cruise to a tropical island. As your body gets healthier, perhaps your adventure will be rediscovering your sexuality or taking up a sport you had previously given up.

In addition to supplying variety and making you feel good about yourself, adventures play a crucial role in the success of your weight management program by providing you incentives. Plan adventures as ways to reward yourself for staying on your food and exercise plans. Since rates of weight loss are so unpredictable, it is dangerous to focus all your attention on the numbers on the scale. Instead, congratulate yourself for keeping on track for two months, or trying a new vegetable every week for a month, or for working out at the gym for an extra thirty minutes.

Adventures Exercise

Make three separate lists of adventures you would like to have: one of small adventures, one for mid-sized adventures, and one for large ones. Brainstorm without reserve for a few minutes, then go back to each list and prioritize the ideas. Which ones would you like to undertake just to add variety to your life? Which ones would work well as incentives to keep on track with your goals for the California Wine Country Diet program? Post your final prioritized lists where you will see them everyday to remind yourself to do them and to motivate you toward your goals.

Remember that whenever you step outside of the comfort zone of what you know, you will be faced with an undetermined outcome. You have the choice to look at this uncertainty with either anxiety or excitement. In Part II you will be starting on the California Wine Country Diet program itself. You will be encouraged to try new foods and methods of preparation. So, start now with viewing the California Wine Country Diet as an exciting adventure. This attitude will enable you to look at your experience in a positive way rather than as "just another diet" that may or may not work. An optimistic perspective will also help you see the challenges you inevitably will encounter as stepping stones in that adventure, rather than as stumbling blocks that can stop your progress or cause you to lose track of your goals.

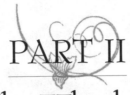

PART II
The Wheel in Motion

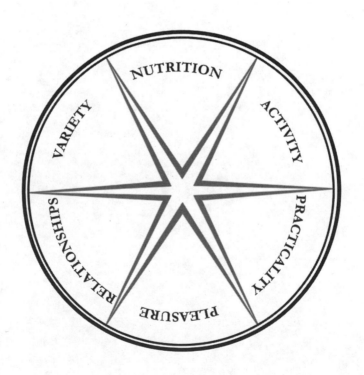

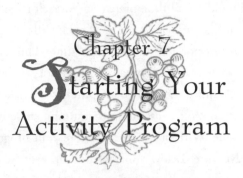

Chapter 7
Starting Your Activity Program

"You can lose weight on any kind of a diet; the trick is to keep it off by finding a healthful way of eating you can live with and a regimen of physical activity you can stick to."
—*Andrew Weil, M.D., and Rosie Daley,*
authors of The Healthy Kitchen

Now that you have examined the six aspects of the Wheel of Weight-Management, it is truly time to put the wheel and yourself into motion. Part II of the *California Wine Country Diet* is where you implement both the nutritional and activity aspects of the program. In order to make this a program that you can follow for the rest of your life, it is essential that each day you also include the other four aspects of the Wheel: practicality, pleasure, relationships, and variety. Chapter 7 will focus on your activity program. Chapters 8, 9, 11, and 12 will introduce you to the nutritional program, the daily meal plans, wine and pleasure foods, and the restaurants of the California wine country. So let's move!

Preparing for Your Activity Program

Beginning an activity program can be quite an undertaking if you are not used to exercising regularly. What do I wear? Could I get hurt? How much water should I be drinking? The questions, large and small, start piling up. When you face any new experience, whether it is a vacation to an exotic country or trying a new restaurant, you face the unknown, but you also face a choice about how to approach uncertainty. You can consider your new undertaking an adventure or a stressful situation you have to get through. That is why as you begin your activity program, you should spend time preparing yourself to make it enjoyable because what you find enjoyable, you will stick with.

The key, as just pointed out, is preparation. Think about how you get ready to go on a trip. You probably would not set foot out the door unless you had scheduled the time to go, purchased a ticket, and packed a suitcase of clothes and other essentials. Beginning an activity program is very much the same. With proper preparation, your program can also be an enjoyable adventure. Below you will find an exercise checklist. Take time now to carefully consider each item and the discussion that accompanies it. Check off the items you have already prepared for or completed.

Exercise Checklist

1. _____ *I have made a commitment to being a lifetime exerciser.*

Think back to the first tier of the practicality pyramid: Cooperating. It is essential when you begin your physical activity program to have the agreement of both your logical conscious self and your emotional basic self. It is one thing to know rationally that you need to exercise to lose weight and keep it off. It is another thing to accept emotionally that you are becoming a lifetime exerciser. Without this internal cooperation, there is a good chance your commitment to exercise will not last. Your conscious self may come up with all sorts of things you need to do that are more important than exercising. Your basic self may get bored and want to do something that it considers more fun. Reassuring yourself that you are a lifetime exerciser, *even though you may not be at this moment,* will help exercise become a natural and indispensable part of your daily life.

2. _____ *I have completed the PAR-Q Test.*

This test, introduced in Chapter 2, makes sure you are physically prepared to exercise. If you have not already done so, complete this questionnaire and follow through with your doctor if so indicated.

3. _____ *I assessed my baseline fitness level and know how much physical activity I need to do to lose weight.*

The International Physical Activity Questionnaire in Chapter 2 gave you your baseline fitness level: inactive, minimally active, or very active. Also in Chapter 2, you learned that to facilitate weight loss you must daily undertake 60-90 minutes of moderate physical activity. In other words, you should now know where you currently are and where you need to be in terms of physical activity.

4. _____ *I identified my barriers to exercise and solutions for how to overcome them.*

Look back to Chapter 2 where you identified your potential barriers to exercise. If you have not already done so, list some potential solutions to these barriers and implement them. If one of your barriers is that you feel you do not have enough time for exercise, think about breaking your exercise into smaller chunks or forgoing some other activity to make room for exercise. Remind yourself that it is not that you cannot afford the time to exercise but more that you cannot afford not to exercise.

5. _____ *I have chosen types of exercise that I enjoy.*

In the activity pyramid introduced in Chapter 2, the tier with the most choices is Aerobic Activity. It is important to choose aerobic activities that you enjoy whether they are individual, group oriented, or competitive. Review the list below and circle those aerobic activities that appeal to you. This is a good place to bring pleasure, relationships, and variety into your physical activity and your life. Remember, just because you have never done something does not mean you cannot do it.

Aerobic Dancing	Bicycling
Energetic Dancing	Brisk Walking
Stair Climbing	Skating
Cross-Country Skiing	Vigorous Ball Sports
Running/Jogging	Swimming
Upper Body Ergometer	Water Aerobics
Other _____	

6. _____ *I have my support team.*

Support for your exercise program is crucial, especially if you are a beginning exerciser. Having a support team will most likely reinforce the structure you will need to make exercise a part of your life. This can be a friend to exercise with, a spouse who takes over your responsibilities temporarily while you exercise, a fitness trainer, or your physician.

Think of those who will encourage you and those who will hold you accountable for sticking to your exercise program. Even your dog can be a member of your team. There is nothing like that eager face waiting for a walk to get you out the door! Be sure to let people know you consider them a part of your support team so they can be there for you. Circle possible support team members below. The more the better!

Spouse/Partner	Dog	Friend
Fitness Trainer	Doctor	Neighbor
Coworker	Sibling	Children

Others _____

7. _____ *I will do my physical activities in these locations (circle):*

Health Club*	Neighborhood
Community Center*	Home
Park	High School Track
Online Fitness Program	Other _____

8. _____ *I have scheduled my exercise. I will begin on*
_____ *(date).*

Remember that it takes about six months for a new behavior to be "locked in," so the more you are able to schedule your exercise, the better chance of successfully making exercise a long-term part of your life. Get out your date book, calendar, palm pilot, whatever, and write in the days

For these choices, do you need to sign up for a membership, or enroll in a class? Now is the time to do so.

and times you will exercise, in ink. If you have days that are packed with other activities, see if you can reschedule one or two, or work in ten-minute bouts of exercise over the course of a day instead of one long one. It is important that you keep these appointments with yourself, just as you would with your doctor or hairdresser, and let nothing interfere. If your program involves exercising with a friend, be sure to coordinate schedules so you have that extra accountability.

You do not need to schedule sixty to ninety minutes a day right from the start. This is a goal. If you have not exercised very much in the past, you will work up to it gradually. If you are only able to walk for ten minutes before getting winded, that is ok. Congratulate yourself on that accomplishment! Then increase your exercise by no more than 10 percent per week. For example if you are able to walk briskly for ten minutes a day the first week, increase the exercise period by one minute the next week. (Your exercise period will be eleven minutes a day during the second week.)

9. _____ *I have the equipment I need to begin my*
exercise program.

Proper equipment ensures your comfort and accountability, and it can even help you monitor your progress. For your chosen activity, make sure you have adequate clothing for that activity, including the proper athletic shoes, and changes of clothes so you always have clean ones on hand. Look over the following list to see what else you might need to properly undertake your chosen exercise program:

- Comfort equipment: Proper clothing and shoes, water bottle, sun screen

- Accountability equipment: calendar/appointment book, health club membership, class enrollment

- Progress and monitoring equipment: Heart rate monitor, watch with stopwatch, pedometer, speedometer, exercise log

- Other _____

10. _____ *I am practicing strategies that reinforce my exercise environment.*

If you have already completed the first nine parts of the checklist, you have already begun programming your environment for exercise. But there also are other small strategies you can use to reinforce your commitment to exercise. For example, make sure you put out your exercise clothes the night before, or call your friend to confirm your exercise date and time. You may want to consider self-rewards, both short term and long term, to motivate your commitment to exercise. Short-term rewards might be treating yourself to a special activity, such as a massage or your favorite pleasure food, after completing your exercise for the week. A long-term reward might be splurging on a new item of clothing after you have consistently walked thirty minutes a day for a month. Each kind of reward is important in reinforcing your exercise environment, so take a moment now to list some short-term and long-term rewards.

11. _____ *I know my fluid needs.*

The ideal amount of fluid intake while exercising is influenced by many variables: how heavily you perspire, the intensity of the activity, and even weather conditions. Drinking enough water is crucial, for dehydration not only can cause discomfort, it can be deadly. The following tips will help you keep yourself well hydrated during exercise:

- Avoid exercise in very hot weather; put it off until cooler parts of the day.

- When exercising out of doors, wear light-colored clothing to reflect heat.

- Drink extra fluids after exercise, rather than before or during, if incontinence is a problem.

- Do not voluntarily limit fluid intake if taking diuretics or laxatives; talk to your doctor if you have a problem with night-time incontinence that is related to medications you are taking.

- *Do not ignore feeling thirsty!*

Workout Hydration Schedule[1]

- Before workout: Two to three hours before you work out, drink 16 to 24 ounces of water

- During workout: Drink 6 to 12 ounces every 15 to 20 minutes

- After workout: Within one hour, drink 2 cups of water for every pound of weight loss. (Weigh yourself before and after exercise.)

For exercise bouts of 60 minutes or less, your fluid of choice should be water. If you are exercising for more than 60 minutes, especially in the heat or at a vigorous intensity, consider a sports drink. The advantage of sports drinks is that they not only replace fluid but also electrolytes, like sodium and potassium that are lost through perspiration. Look for sports drinks that contain no more than 8 percent carbohydrate, as higher concentrations can lead to stomach cramping.

Implementing Your Activity Program

In Chapter 2, you were introduced to the California Wine Country Diet activity pyramid, which contains the seven components of an activity program: Activities of Daily Living, Aerobic Activity, Balance and Flexibility, Strength Training, Anaerobic Activity, and Rest. It is now time to further address each of these components so that you can design your own personal physical activity program.

First Tier of the Activity Pyramid: Activities of Daily Living

The first tier covers the exercise you get from going about the activities of normal daily life: climbing stairs, house cleaning, playing with your kids, walking the corridors at work, and so on. Although these types of activities normally do not do much to truly improve your fitness level, they all burn calories and so can affect your weight. Even fidgeting, like jiggling your left foot or tapping you hand on your desk or constantly squirming in your chair, will burn calories: up to 350 extra calories a day![2] This is not to say that if you just start jiggling your left foot you will lose weight, but rather it indicates how the smallest sustained increase in activities of daily living can profoundly affect energy balance.*

Review the table below to see how simple changes in the level of activity in your daily routine can increase your caloric expenditure:

High-ADL Activity	Calories**	Low-ADL Activity	Calories**
Getting up and changing the TV	3	Using the remote	0.6
Talking on the phone for 30 minutes, pacing	162	Talking on the phone for 30 minutes, sitting	42
Manually opening garage door	3	Using garage door opener	0.25
Moderate housework (scrubbing, sweeping, vacuuming) for 1 hour	152	Hiring a housekeeper	0.0
15 minutes chopping vegetables	13	Buying pre-chopped vegetables	0.0
30 minutes gardening plus 30 minutes mowing with a push mower	360	Hiring a lawn service	0.0
Walking the dog for 30 minutes	125	Letting the dog out the back door	2.0
Parking at the back of the lot and walking 1–2 minutes to the store	8	Parking close to the store	0.3
Taking the stairs three flights	45	Taking the elevator 3 flights	1.0
Total calories used	871	Total calories used	46.15

By doing the activities in the High-ADL list just once throughout the week, you would use an additional 825 extra calories per week, which could result in a twelve pound weight loss per year.

List below three ways you can increase your ADLs:

1.

2.

3.

* Can a former couch potato become a fidgeter? It is unlikely since this is an inherited trait. Obese people who lose weight tend to still move less, and fidgeters who gain weight tend to still fidget. However, if you are sedentary to begin with, making a conscious effort to increase your activities of daily living can greatly affect your weight-loss potential.

** Based on an individual weighing 150 lbs. Add or subtract 10 percent for each 15 lbs over or under 150 lbs.

Second Tier of the Activity Pyramid: Aerobic Activity

If you are new to exercise, you may not realize that how you begin and end your exercise period are important elements of safe workouts. These are called the "warm-up" and "cool-down" periods, and you must not skip them. They are part of every proper exercise routine, whether it is aerobic or not. With aerobic activity in particular, however, there are some other considerations that will help you have a more enjoyable and beneficial time exercising. These considerations are the focus of this section.

Warm-Up and Cool-Down Periods

A proper warm-up before exercise helps to raise your core body temperature, loosening your muscle fibers and thus preparing them for the impending exercise session. Without a proper warm-up, you increase your risk of muscle damage. The basic way of warming up is to do your intended activity (i.e. walking, cycling, swimming) for five minutes at an easy intensity. Follow this with five minutes of muscle-specific stretching.

The cool-down period helps your blood flow return to normal and facilitates the removal of metabolic waste products out of the blood, thereby diminishing muscle soreness. The cool-down routine is similar to the warm-up period—five minutes of easy activity and five minutes of muscle-specific stretching.

Frequency, Intensity, Time (FIT)

After your warm-up period, you will begin to increase your exercise intensity until it reaches the aerobic level. But there are three aspects to this intense activity period that determine its health payoff: frequency, intensity, and time, or FIT, for short. Let us take a look at each aspect individually and then put them together to illustrate an effective exercise program.

Frequency

For weight loss, you need to exercise five to six days per week. If you are a beginning exerciser, think of this frequency as a goal to achieve, not something you should initially try to accomplish. Begin by exercising three days a week, with at least one day of rest in between exercise days. As you improve your fitness level and stamina, begin to increase your days of exercise until you comfortably meet the minimum of five to six days per week.

Intensity

The intensity of your workout refers to how hard you are exerting yourself. People who are just beginning an exercise program often think they need to push themselves until they are huffing and puffing to get any training effect. Granted, you do need to exercise more vigorously than a casual walk, but not so vigorously that you are breathless. How do you know if you are exerting yourself too hard or not hard enough? Fortunately, there are two tried and true methods for finding a proper intensity level for aerobic fitness: Training Heart Rate and the Talk-Sing Rule.

1. Your Training Heart Rate can be predicted using the following formula:[3]

Training Heart Rate = Maximum Heart Rate x 60 percent to 90 percent.

Maximum Heart Rate is defined as 220 minus your age. Your actual Maximum Heart Rate can deviate by 10 to 12 beats per minute from this equation, but this formula serves as a good prediction. Use 60 percent if you are sedentary, and up to 90 percent if you are more fit. For example, a 45-year-old sedentary woman's training heart rate would be (220-45) x 60 percent = 105 beats per minute. Take this number and divide it by six to get a 10-second pulse. This woman would have a 10-second pulse of 17.5, or 17 to 18 beats every 10 seconds.

The easiest place to take your pulse is by placing two fingers of one hand lightly on one side of the throat or, as some people prefer, on the inside of your wrist. During aerobic activity, take your pulse every five minutes or so to see if you are at your Training Heart Rate. If you are above that rate, slow down your pace; if you are below, pick it up.

If you have a heart-rate monitor, your heart rate will be available to you continuously. Many models beep at you if you go above or below your Training Heart Rate. If you take a 10-second pulse, stop and immediately count the number of beats in 10 seconds, rather than trying to count while exercising.

Calculate your Training Heart Rate:

220 - _____ (your age) x _____ % = _____ beats per minute.

Take this number _____ ÷ 6 = _____ (10-second pulse)

2. An even easier method of estimating a proper exertion level is using the Talk-Sing Rule. You should be exercising at a rate where you are able to easily stay in a conversation without becoming breathless, but are not easily able to sing. If you need to catch your breath with every sentence, slow down! If you can hum your favorite tune, you need to pick up the pace.

Time

Time of exercise refers to the duration in minutes at which you sustain the intensity of your workout. The USDA *Dietary Guidelines 2005* recommends 60 to 90 minutes of moderate-intensity exercise a day for weight loss. As mentioned previously, this is a goal, not the level at which you start your program, especially if you have led a sedentary lifestyle.

In addition, studies have shown that several short workouts over the course of a day can be as effective as one long workout, so you do you not have to devote a solid hour and a half block of your time to exercise. If you have two 15-minute breaks at work, for example, you could walk during these breaks and then do an additional 30 minutes of exercise after work. You do not have to do only aerobic exercise for the entire 60-90 minutes. This time period could include your (high) ADLs, strength training, and flexibility sessions as well. However, the more aerobic exercise you do, the sooner you will see weight-loss results.

Rate of Progression

How fast you are able to progress from being inactive to active depends on many things including your health status, age, and family support, just to name a few. The key is to make gradual yet consistent efforts to increase your frequency, intensity, and time of exercise.[4, 5] The following table serves as a guideline for your rate of progression. The intensity is figured by your Training Heat Rate. First look at your fitness level, which you figured out from the International Physical Activity Questionnaire in Chapter 2, then look to the corresponding Frequency, Intensity, and Time for your exercise:

Weight-Loss Guidelines for Exercise by Fitness Level			
Current Fitness Level:	*Inactive*	*Minimally Active*	*Very Active*
Days per week of exercise:	3 or less	3-4	5+
Intensity (% Max Heart Rate):	60%-70%	70%-80%	80%-90%
Minutes of exercise per day:	10-20	15-45	60-90
Number of weeks at each level:	4-6	12-20	6 months+

Third Tier of the Activity Pyramid
Balance

As discussed in Chapter 2, balance is an important component of overall fitness. Having good balance has been shown to reduce such conditions as chronic knee pain, low-back pain, arm numbness, and acute ankle sprains.[6] The good news is that balance can be improved with regular exercise, whether it is aerobic, strength training, or any other form of exercise that challenges your balance.

Examples of specific balance exercises include:

- Balance equipment (wobble board, rocker board, balance sandals, BOSU ball)
- Yoga
- Tai chi
- Strength training (especially free weights)
- Standing exercises (like the one mentioned below)
- Walking on uneven surfaces (beach, grass)

Evaluating Your Balance

There is a simple single-leg stance test that you can do to evaluate your balance.[7] In doing this initially, place a table or chair next to you to hold on to in case you lose your balance. As you get better at this exercise, you will be able to do it without the support of a table or chair.

Either barefoot or wearing comfortable shoes or athletic shoes, raise one foot a few inches straight up off the ground without touching it to your other foot or leg, called the "support" foot or leg in these instructions. Keep your eyes open, and you can look around normally.

1. Count off seconds, and note the longest time you can maintain this position. As soon as the raised foot touches your support foot or leg, the floor, or anything else that could give it support, or you are hopping, consider the exercise over. Or if you lose your balance and have to reach out for support, consider the exercise over.

2. Practice this exercise until you can maintain your balance on one foot for 30 seconds straight.

3. Once you can do this exercise for 30 seconds, try practicing it with your eyes open but gazed fixed at one spot straight ahead. When you have mastered this variation of the exercise, practice it again until you can do it for 30 seconds with your eyes closed.

There is no specific recommendation for frequency or duration of balance exercises, except to incorporate them regularly into your exercise program.

Flexibility

Like balance, flexibility is often neglected, yet it can have a profound impact on your overall fitness. One of the easiest ways to improve your flexibility is with regular stretching. Incorporating five minutes of muscle-specific stretching to your warm-up and cool-down periods is an important part of keeping your muscles flexible and reducing your risk of injury. Adding a separate and fuller stretching routine will even further enhance your level of flexibility.

How to Stretch

There are several methods for improving flexibility, but the static method appears to be most practical, with little risk of injury or pain.[8] In this method, you slowly stretch out your muscle and then hold it at full stretch for a brief time, as follows:

1. Begin with a 4-5 minute warm up of light exercise.

2. Slowly stretch the muscle just used until you feel a mild tension, then stop.

3. Hold the stretch without bouncing for 10-30 seconds. Remember to relax and breathe during the stretching.

4. When the tightness of the stretch starts to subside, this means the muscle is relaxing and you can now move a little deeper into the stretch, just until you feel the mild tension again. Hold this new position without bouncing for 30-60 seconds, relaxing and breathing through the stretch.

5. Repeat with each major muscle group of the body.

The most important time to stretch is immediately after exercise because the muscles are naturally most flexible at this time. A good resource for illustrations of stretching exercises is *Stretching* by Bob Anderson (www.shelterpub.com).

Fourth Tier of the Activity Pyramid: Strength Training

The goal of strength training is to improve muscle strength and endurance. Significant improvements in muscle function can be made with a consistent 30-minute workout two to three times per week. Your program should be progressive in nature, which means that you are consistently increasing the amount of weight as you grow more fit, to challenge the muscle group you are working but not so much as to cause injury.

There are three types of strength training:

1. *Isometric:* With isometrics, the muscle contracts against a fixed immovable resistance. Pushing against a wall is an isometric contraction. Each contraction should be held for six seconds using 100 percent of your strength, and repeated 5 to 10 times. The advantages of this method are that they are easy to perform, they can be done anywhere, and they require little time or expense. The disadvantage of isometrics is that it only works for the angle your muscle is working rather than a complete range of motion.

2. *Isotonic:* This type of strength training involves the contraction of the muscle against resistance with movement, such as occurs with weight machines, free-weights, and calisthenics such as push-ups or sit-ups. As

your strength improves over time, you add more weight or repetitions to your routine. If you choose this route, be sure to make an appointment with a fitness trainer who can teach proper form for lifting, as well as design a program with your specific goals in mind. If you are a health club member, this service is often free. Exercises like Pilates or Power Yoga also incorporate this type of strength training, plus flexibility and balance.

3. *Isokinetic:* These types of exercises are those in which the speed of muscular contraction is constant but the resistance to the muscular contraction is proportional to the force of contraction. In other words, the harder you push or pull, the more resistance you will feel. Isokinetic training is most useful in neuromuscular rehabilitation and for training elite athletes.

In this program, we will concentrate on isotonic strength training because it offers a variety of choices and numerous benefits. The following guidelines are for standard weight training:

1. Warm-up and cool-down periods. These periods can consist of either walking (as on a treadmill) for five or ten minutes before and after lifting, or lifting a lower amount of weight for one easy set to begin your routine.

2. During your routine, perform the lifts slowly. If you lift weight quickly, you will be using your momentum or gravity to move the weight, not your muscle alone. This not only minimizes the improvement to your muscle but can also cause injury. Studies have shown that a moderate velocity lift and lowering of one to two seconds in each direction has the most beneficial effect on muscle performance and strength gains.[9, 10, 11] Take a two-second to three-second rest before the next repetition. You may want to count out loud when strength training at first to help you set the pace: "Lift (one, two), lower (one, two), rest (one, two, three)…"

3. You should be able to lift the intended weight 8–12 times in good form at the rate mentioned above. If you cannot lift the weight eight times in good form, lower the amount of weight. If you can lift the weight more than twelve times in good form, increase the amount of weight.

4. Take a one-minute to three-minute rest between sets. A set is one round of eight to twelve repetitions in good form.

5. Work up to three sets of each exercise.

6. To maximize strength gains, work large muscle groups such as the upper legs, upper arms, hips, chest, and back before smaller muscle

groups like the lower arms, abdomen, and lower legs.

7. Do not forget to breathe! Most people want to hold their breath during lifts. Unfortunately, this can put pressure on the chest, preventing blood from leaving the muscles. During the lift, exhale. During the lowering, inhale. An easy rule to remember this breathing pattern is "EXercise (lift) EXhale."

8. Progress gradually yet consistently. When you can complete more than twelve repetitions in good form, add more weight but no more than 10 percent of your previous weight or the amount that will get you back to being able to complete between eight and twelve repetitions in good form. This gradual weight increase will force your muscles to continually work harder and thus improve muscle strength, size, and tone.

How Not to Get Huge

"Bulking up" is a concern of many women who begin strength training. But this masculinization of the physique is usually not a problem. The good news for women is they have on average one-tenth the amount of testosterone as men, which is the hormone responsible for muscle size. Granted, with weight training, a woman's muscle tone will improve, so her muscles will feel firmer and appear more defined, but it takes a certain type of lifting to increase muscle size. The program recommended here will not significantly increase muscle size. Other measures you can take if you are concerned with this issue include:

- Do your aerobic workout after strength training
- Rest between sets
- Do not lift to the point of "muscle fatigue," which means doing sets until you absolutely cannot physically complete another repetition.

Fifth Tier of the Activity Pyramid: Anaerobic Activity

Anaerobic exercise can be incorporated into your aerobic session two or three times a week. One way to do this is to exercise in what are called "intervals." If you are walking for aerobic exercise, for example, then to add an anaerobic interval to your routine, simply walk faster or increase your pace to a jog for one minute or less every five minutes throughout your walk. To gauge when you have reached an anaerobic level, just pay attention: You should feel winded and ready to slow down at the end of the anaerobic interval. Follow up this interval with a slow recovery period that is at least three times as long as the interval. A walking interval program would look something like this:

- Warm up with 5 minutes of easy walking.
- Increase your pace to training heart-rate level for 5 minutes.
- Then speed walk or jog for 30 seconds.
- Drop back to walking at your training heart-rate level for the next 2 minutes.
- Pick up the pace with a speed walk or jog for 30 seconds.
- Drop back to the training heart-rate level for the next 2 minutes.
- Continue this interval schedule for a set portion or the rest of your aerobic workout.

As your fitness level improves, you can increase the level of intensity for your interval training in at least three ways:

1. Increase the duration of each interval segment, or

2. Keep the interval time the same but increase the *intensity* of the segment, or

3. Keep the duration and intensity of the segments the same but increase the number of interval segments you perform during your routine.

Do not change the duration, intensity, or number of anaerobic segments more often than once a week. The key is to progress slowly and gradually—too rapid a progression can cause injury.

Top of the Activity Pyramid: Rest

The last tier of the California Wine Country Diet activity pyramid is rest. After any workout routine, your muscles will need time to replace proteins and energy stores they used during the exercise. If you do not give your muscles adequate time to recover, your muscle size could actually decrease, lowering your metabolism as a result. Not giving muscles enough rest can also cause exercise "burnout," which would put a definite damper on your weight-loss progress.

Another term for not getting enough muscle rest is overtraining. Your body is the arbiter of what constitutes overtraining for you. These very physical signs include:

- Mild leg soreness, general achiness
- Resting pulse 5-10 beats per minute higher than normal
- Pain in muscles and joints
- Washed-out feeling, tired, drained, lack of energy
- Sudden drop in ability to run "normal" distances or times
- Insomnia
- Headaches
- Inability to relax, twitchy, fidgety
- Insatiable thirst, dehydration
- Lowered resistance to common illnesses: colds, sore throat, etc.

Think of rest as preparing your muscles for your next exercise session. These pointers will also help ensure that you allow enough time for your muscles to adequately rest and recover:

- Get plenty of sleep.
- Allow at least one day "off" between similar types of workouts. Choose one day per week for nothing but rest, with no exercise except the activities of daily living.
- After an aerobic exercise bout of 60 minutes or more, follow up with a high carbohydrate food or beverage to replenish glycogen stores.
- Drink plenty of fluids, to the point where your urine is pale yellow or lighter.
- Keep your exercise routine varied in order to not overuse muscle groups.

Maintaining Your Activity Program

Preparing for and implementing an exercise routine is one thing; maintaining a lifelong program is a whole different challenge. It takes up to six months for exercise to become engrained into your lifestyle. If you are not used to exercising on a regular basis, chances are there will be some point during that initial six months that your body, or your basic self or your conscious self, will rebel at all this exercise. Consciously or subconsciously, you may start looking for ways to slip back into your old ways. Even elite athletes battle with this desire to not exercise so much, but what stops them from quitting is having built-in tactics to keep their bodies and environment motivated for exercise. There are numerous strategies you can use. The key is finding the ones that work for you. Some tried-and-true strategies follow.

Track Your Progress

Progress monitoring is a powerful tool to enhance motivation because it clearly shows your improvement over time. The best way to monitor your progress is with an activity log. In your log, jot down the date, what activity you did, and for how long you did it. Additional notes could include the estimated number of calories expended, your current weight, your resting heart rate, and your feelings and goals. Over time, your log will reveal the clear results of your dedication to good health: improving fitness levels and dropping weight. That kind of irrefutable testimonial can keep you on track with your exercise program or motivate you to a higher level of intensity.

The key to maintaining a log is to select the style of log that fits your needs and provides the kind of information that is meaningful to you. A log can be as simple as a spiral-bound notebook or as elaborate as a special leather covered journal. You can even use your desk calendar or date book. You can start a separate log for strength training if you go to a health club.

You can go online to a Web site (there are many) where you can enter your exercise data and they will do the rest, such as tracking your calories expended, miles walked, and minutes used.[12] Give keeping a log a try because you may find that tracking your progress provides just the right motivation for you to keep going with your exercise program.

Rewards

We live in a society where we expect instant results to keep us going. When it comes to exercise, we often feel a need to see results quickly because of all the time and effort we are investing. Unfortunately, many of the benefits of exercise are not seen overnight, but over time. This delayed gratification is why creating other rewards for yourself is important. Rewards give us a short-term benefit to pull us through until we begin to see the long-term benefits. By working incentives into your exercise program, you can increase your level of commitment. Choose incentives that will reinforce your resolve to exercise such as:

- A new CD for your Walkman
- A massage
- A new piece of exercise clothing
- A subscription to a fitness magazine

You also may want to have some small rewards to get you through the week and save the bigger rewards for reaching pre-determined fitness goals. For example, you could indulge in a bubble bath at the end of the week and schedule a massage for the end of the month. The key is to find rewards that work for you, and to schedule them in your activity log to motivate you toward your goal.

Create a realistic activity schedule

Over-commitment is a recipe for failure. Even a temporary failure can increase the risk that you will eventually discontinue your overall exercise program. So start by doing what you can do, and no more. If three days a week of exercise is all you can comfortably manage, fine! By keeping exercise a positive part of your life and setting realistic goals, you will create a recipe for success.

Stay injury free

Becoming injured not only dampens your emotional commitment to exercise, but it can be a serious physical setback as well. Even with the best planning, safeguarding, and self-nurturing, injury can happen. Preventing an injury can be as simple as listening to your body when it is telling you that you are doing too much.

Prevention also involves adequately warming up, stretching, and cooling down.

The more you exercise, the more you will be able to distinguish between the type of pain that is due to your body getting used to exercise and the pain that is due to injury. A common pain that occurs when using your body in a way it is not used to is sore muscles. Sore muscles are typically felt on both sides of the body and usually arise 24 hours after a workout. Then the stiffness and soreness slowly subside.

Pain from an actual injury typically occurs only in one area and tends to be sharper and more acute. If you feel this type of pain, back off. Do not be shy about telling your exercise partner to slow down or taking a break from an exercise class if you feel something is not right. Attempting to push through an injury type of pain can only make it worse and prolong your recovery.

However, even if you do experience an injury, you often do not have to stop exercising completely. Say, for example, that you got a shin splint from jogging. You could switch to swimming or cycling, and you could continue with your strength training, flexibility sessions, and balance routine. In other words, avoid the types of exercises that aggravate your injury.

It's All Good

Making the commitment to change from being a non-exerciser to an exerciser takes a lot of motivation, patience, and perseverance. Fortunately, many of the tools we have discussed will help you make a smooth transition, and one that has a sense of excitement and even adventure.

Use these tools as you see fit, but always remember that your goal of being a more active person is multifaceted. You will more fully engage in life's varieties, increase your pleasure as you try new things and feel better, get fit, lose weight, and more easily keep that weight off for a lifetime.

Chapter 8
Getting Ready to Start the Daily Meal Plans

"The pleasures of the table—that lovely old-fashioned phrase—depict food as an art form, as a delightful part of civilized life. In spite of food fads, fitness programs, and health concerns, we must never lose sight of a beautifully conceived meal."
— *Julia Child*

You are now at the point where many diet books begin—the introduction of the meal plans for losing weight. How are you feeling? Excited? Optimistic? Impatient? Anxious? "Can't we just keep talking about the theory?" "I want to start today." "I can't start until after the holidays." All of these are perfectly normal feelings and thoughts. You probably have some of them running around in your head right now. Before beginning anything new, it is natural to feel anxious. Just remember that another aspect of anxiety is *excitement*.

In choosing the California Wine Country Diet, you have chosen a program that is based on the latest scientific research and the experience of thousands of years of healthy traditional diets. You will be eating and drinking fresh, seasonal foods and beverages. You will get to experience the recipes of some of the California wine country's finest chefs in the comfort of your own home. And, you will be attending to all six aspects of the Wheel of Weight-Management, which will ensure an enjoyable experience that will lead to the creation of your own unique blueprint for long-term weight maintenance.

Keep your focus on these positive thoughts as you go through the Daily Meal Plans—Starting Checklist, which follows. If there are any items you cannot check off yet, take the time now to handle them. The more prepared you are, the easier starting will be.

Daily Meal Plans—Starting Checklist

1. _____ *I have made a commitment to embrace a lifestyle that will lead to reaching and maintaining a healthy weight.*

While you may have picked up *The California Wine Country Diet* in the hopes of finding a quick-fix diet, I am sure, it is obvious by now that what we are really talking about is a lifestyle change—one that will get you off the diet roller coaster once and for all. As we talked about in Chapter 7, Starting Your Activity Program, this long-term commitment is one that must be embraced by both your logical, conscious self and your emotional, basic self.

To meet your conscious self's need to mentally understand your goal, this chapter will present technical information to prepare you for starting the Daily Meal Plans of the California Wine Country Diet. If your basic self starts to get bored and impatient with this chapter, assure it that fun and adventure are just around the corner with later chapters talking about wine, pleasure foods, and a tour of the California wine country.

2. _____ *I have asked for support from those I live with and those with whom I have daily contact.*

It is essential to talk with the people you live with before starting the Daily Meal Plans since these changes will affect everyone. If your family wants to be on the program with you, then educate them about it and have them figure out what calorie level they will be on. For those who do not or should not join you completely—for example, children—you can introduce them to many of the same foods you eat while still fixing their favorites. With friends and coworkers, ask for the kind of support you would like from them: "Please don't offer me cookies," or "Let's go to a restaurant where I can get a salad for lunch."

3. _____ *I have cleaned out and organized my eating and cooking environment so that I am ready to start the Daily Meal Plans.*

Clearing out your kitchen and food storage areas is an important aspect of getting ready. Go through your cupboards and refrigerator, and get rid of those foods that will not be part of your new eating style. While you will have a certain number of calories each day for pleasure foods, do you really want to spend these limited calories on a handful of chips? If you are living with others who want these types of foods, put them in a special place that will be out of sight for you. Getting your kitchen organized now will make food preparation easier once you begin the Daily Meal Plans in Chapter 9.

4. _____ *I have gathered the utensils, dishes, glasses, and table linen that I will need.*

Make sure that you have a collection of measuring utensils conveniently at hand, including: multiple sets of measuring spoons, several measuring cups, and a food scale. In the process of educating yourself about portion sizes, it will be very important to weigh and measure your food.

As we talked about in Chapter 3, small plates and tall thin glasses have a positive effect on feeling satisfied with smaller amounts of food and drink. Have a bowl or basket out on the counter ready for the fruit you are going to purchase. Perhaps it is time to buy some new plates or table linen to celebrate the beginning of this program and to help you appreciate the wonderful meals you are going to prepare.

5. _____ *I have a collection of storage containers.*

Having storage containers of different sizes can be crucial in preventing overeating and making your new choices easier to carry out. Be sure to have microwave-safe containers for anything you want to reheat. Store what you will not be eating. For example, rather than being tempted by that extra helping that is sitting out on the table or counter, store it, and put it out of sight. Instead of eating everything on your plate, remind yourself that you can use leftovers as the basis for another meal, making that meal's preparation easier and faster.

6. _____ *I have the cookware and kitchen appliances that I will need.*

The recipes in the California Wine Country Diet require some basic kitchen equipment. You will need a set of pots and pans with at least one or two frying pans. You will need a 9" x 12" roasting pan, a baking sheet, a sieve, and a MISTO spray can. Many of the recipes recommend grilling, which can be done either inside or outside. If you are unable to grill, you can always use the broiler. Appliances you should have on hand include a toaster, microwave, blender, hand-held blender, and food processor. If you want to make the COPIA sorbet recipe, you will need an ice-cream maker.

7. _____ *I know where I can purchase the food items that I will need.*

Now is a good time to visit local stores, co-ops, and farmers' markets to scout out where you will purchase the items needed for the Daily Meal Plans. Look over their herb and spice section, their Asian food section, and their Latin food section. Spend some time reviewing the different oils and vinegars. Where will you get the freshest meat and fish? Where is the best place to get fresh produce? Is there someone at the store who is knowledgeable and willing to help you find unusual items? Do you have a local natural foods store? Where is the best place to purchase wine? If you cannot find items close to where you live, there are excellent online sources, some of which are listed in the Suggested Reading and Resources section at the back of this book.

The more you look around before you actually start the Daily Meal Plans, the easier it will be when you encounter a recipe requiring grape seed oil or Mache or other less familiar food. Remember that discovering and trying out novel foods is part of what will keep this program new and exciting for you.

8. _____ *I am going to start the California Wine Country*
   Diet Daily Meal Plans on _____ (date).

Think about the most opportune time to start the Daily Meal Plans to ensure you get off to a good start: the first of the month, a Monday, after a big event, before a big event. Find a time before your start date to buy the food you will need for the first three days. The shopping list for these three days is in the next chapter. During the first week, you will be given suggestions for all your meals and snacks. If you need or want to eat out or make substitutions, you can do so from the servings list at the end of this chapter.

Determining Your Healthy Weight Range and Calorie Level for Weight Loss

Setting a weight goal can make or break your motivation for weight loss. It is imperative that you set a *realistic* goal. While you might yearn to look like the bodies you see on magazine covers, a healthy weight does not mean achieving a particular physique. Trying to achieve a weight that is too low is the mind-set that has contributed to the epidemic of eating disorders. Your goal for weight loss should be based on what is healthy for you, not on what is considered trendy or fashionable. Realistically, a healthy weight is one that decreases the risks associated with disease. Rather than focusing on a specific weight, you will determine a healthy weight range for you.

There are various methods for determining a healthy weight: height-weight charts, percentage of body fat, and circumference measurements, to name a few. The most utilized measuring tool is Body Mass Index, or BMI. This method is reliable for most people between the ages of nineteen and seventy, except women who are pregnant or breast feeding, competitive athletes, body builders, or chronically ill patients. This is the method we will use, so follow the directions that follow.

Step #1—Determine Your Body Mass Index (BMI)

To find your BMI, look at the BMI chart that follows.[1] Find your height in the left column. Do not guess! Take a tape measure and find your exact height. Many people shrink an inch or so with age, so it is important to know what your current height is. Next, weigh yourself on an accurate scale that you can use throughout the program. Find the value closest to your current weight in the row across the top. Follow the column across and the row down to the point where they meet to find your BMI.

My height is: _____ My weight is: _____

My BMI is: _____

Step #2—Determine Your Healthy Weight Range

Use the BMI chart to determine what your healthy weight range should be. Let me provide an example. Mary is 5 feet, 6 inches tall and weighs 180 pounds. According the BMI Chart, Mary's BMI would be 29. Moving across the row to the left to a BMI of 19 to 24, you will see that her healthy weight range would be 120 to 150 pounds. Find what your healthy weight range is.

My healthy weight range is: _____ to _____ pounds

Step #3—Determine Your Range of Weight Loss

The next step is to subtract your healthy weight range from your current weight to determine how much weight you need to lose to move into your healthy weight range. Using our earlier example, Mary would subtract her healthy weight range of 120 to 150 pounds from her current weight of 180 pounds. She needs to lose from 30 to 60 pounds to be in her healthy weight range.

My current weight _____
less my healthy weight range _____ to _____
equals my range of weight to lose _____ to _____

If you feel overwhelmed by the number of pounds you need to lose to move into the healthy BMI weight range, remember that even a 10 percent reduction in weight can lead to substantial improvements in health.[2]

Body Mass Index (BMI)
Weight in pounds

Height	120	130	140	150	160	170	180	190	200	210	220	230	240	250
4' 6"	29	31	34	36	39	41	43	46	48	52	43	46	48	60
4' 8"	27	29	31	34	36	38	40	43	45	47	49	52	54	56
4' 10"	25	27	29	31	34	36	38	40	42	44	46	48	50	52
5' 0"	23	25	27	29	31	33	35	37	39	41	43	45	47	49
5' 2"	22	24	26	27	29	31	33	35	37	38	40	42	44	46
5' 4"	21	22	24	26	28	29	31	33	34	36	38	40	41	43
5' 6"	19	21	23	24	26	27	29	31	32	34	36	37	39	40
5' 8"	18	20	21	23	24	26	27	29	30	32	34	35	37	38
5' 10"	17	19	20	22	23	24	26	27	29	30	32	33	35	36
6' 0"	16	18	19	20	22	23	24	26	27	28	30	31	33	34
6' 2"	15	17	18	19	21	22	23	24	26	27	28	30	31	32
6' 4"	15	16	17	18	20	21	22	23	24	26	27	28	29	30
6' 6"	14	15	16	17	19	20	21	22	23	24	25	27	28	29
6' 8"	13	14	15	17	18	19	20	21	22	23	24	25	26	28

Key
- Obese (30+)
- Overweight (25-29)
- Healthy weight (Below 25)

If you have 30 or more pounds to lose, it is wise to establish an initial goal for weight loss of 10 percent of your current weight. In Mary's case that would mean a loss of 18 pounds. This does not mean that you should stop with the initial 10 percent weight loss, since long-term health benefits are maximized by moving into your healthy weight range.

Those with more than 30 pounds to lose should complete the following:

My current weight of _____ times 10 percent
equals my initial weight-loss goal of _____ pounds.

Step #4—Determine Your Rate of Weight Loss

Studies of long-term weight loss show that losing weight at a rate of one to two pounds a week is associated with long-term weight-loss success. This rate of loss is equivalent to a 500-calorie to 1,000-calorie daily deficit. This calculation does *not* mean you just need to eat 500 to 1,000 fewer calories per day to lose weight. This deficit is created by a combination of fewer calories in and more calories out. For example, if you eat 500 fewer calories per day than you are currently eating and add 500 calories' worth of exercise to your daily activity, you will have created a 1,000-calorie deficit.

Rate of weight loss per week in pounds	Required calorie deficit per day
1	500
1.5	750
2	1,000

My weekly goal for weight loss is _____ pounds by employing a daily deficit of _____ calories

Step #5—Determine the Number of Weeks to Reach Your Goals

Look to how many pounds you need to lose to reach both your initial goal of a 10 percent weight loss and to reach your healthy BMI goal. With a weight loss rate of one to two pounds a week, look at how long it will take you, realistically, to achieve your goals. If you are losing at a faster pace, you may want to slow down to increase the chance of long-term success. If you are not losing quickly enough, you may want to consider bumping up your exercise a notch or decreasing your calorie intake slightly. Complete the following chart to see how long it will take you to reach your goals at different rates of weight loss.

Number of weeks	@ 1 lb/week	@ 1.5 lbs/week	@ 2 lbs/week
10% goal	_____	_____	_____
Healthy BMI goal	_____	_____	_____

Step #6—Determine Your Current Calorie Intake

Before figuring how many calories you need to eat for weight loss, you need to determine how many calories your body needs to maintain its current weight. From that figure, you create your deficit goal. There are many ways to determine your calorie intake. You can keep a food record for a few days and calculate the calories you are eating by consulting a calorie book. This method can be accurate if you are good at analyzing your portions and have a good calorie book, but it can be tedious. Also, if your food intake is not steady, the result will only reveal a "snapshot" of what you ate for a particular period rather then your normal eating pattern.

An easier method of determining your current calorie intake is by estimation. The simplest way is by taking your current weight in pounds and multiplying it by 12. For example, Mary, who weighs 180 pounds, would estimate that she consumes 2,160 calories per day to maintain her weight (180 pounds x 12). Estimate how many calories you eat to maintain your current weight.

My current weight ＿＿＿＿＿ x 12 equals my estimated intake of ＿＿＿＿＿ calories per day that are needed to maintain my present weight.

Step #7—Determine Your Calorie Intake for Weight Loss

Now comes the moment of reckoning. Calories not only count, they are the bottom line when it comes to weight loss. Remember, you need to create your calorie deficit with a combination of diet and exercise. Plan to have at least 300 calories per day of your deficit come from activity. Consult the Calories Used Per Minute During Physical Activity on the next page to see how many calories are burned in various activities.[3, 4] The remainder will make up your calorie intake for weight loss.

To illustrate this calculation, think of Mary, who determined in Step 6 that she needs approximately 2,200 calories per day to maintain her current weight. If she decides she wants to lose two pounds per week, she needs to create a 1,000-calorie deficit. If she decides to do the minimum 300 calories of additional activity per day, she would need to create the remaining 700-calorie deficit by reducing her caloric intake. By subtracting this 700 from her maintenance calories, she finds she needs a 1,500-calorie intake for weight loss. Determine your calorie goal now.

	Mary's example (based on 2 lbs a week):	My numbers:
Deficit needed to lose		
_____ lbs per week	1,000	_____
Less calories burned in activity	-300	_____
Food deficit calories required	700	_____
Current maintenance calories	2,200	_____
Less food deficit calories	-700	_____
Caloric intake for weight loss:	1,500	_____

It is important that your calorie intake per day not fall below 1,200 calories if you are a woman or 1,400 calories if you are a man, because you need at least that many calories to meet daily nutritional requirements.[5] If your calorie intake falls below these levels, decrease the amount of food deficit calories in the above calculation and/or increase the calories you plan to burn in activities. Adjust these amounts until the bottom line, caloric intake for weight loss, matches or exceeds the 1,200 or 1,400 calories required by your body.

Calories Used Per Minute During Physical Activity

Moderate Physical Activity	Calories Used Per Minute
Hiking	6.0
Light gardening/yard work	5.5
Dancing	5.5
Golf (walking and carrying clubs)	5.5
Bicycling	
10 mph	7.0
<10 mph	5.5
Walking (level road, 17 min/mile)	4.5
Strength training (general light workout)	3.5
Stretching	3.0
Swimming (25 yards per minute)	6.0

Vigorous Physical Activity	Calories Used Per Minute
Running/jogging	
12 min/mile	10.0
10 min/mile	12.5
8.5 min/mile	14.5
Bicycling	
11 mph	8.0
12 mph	10.0
Swimming (50 yards per minute)	12.5
Aerobics	11.0
Walking	
Level road, 13 min/mile	7.5
Uphill, 17 min/mile	8 to 15.0
Heavy yard work (chopping wood)	7.5
Strength training (vigorous effort)	7.5
Basketball (vigorous)	7.5
Stair climbing	8.0
Rowing machine	14.0
Skipping rope (vigorous)	13.0

Step #8—Determining Your California Wine Country Daily Meal Plans

The California Wine Country Diet has three levels of calorie values in its meal plans: 1,200, 1,600, or 2,000 calories a day. If your ideal caloric intake for weight loss (as determined in Step # 7) does not fit exactly into one of these plans, choose the plan that is the closest. In our example, Mary would start with Plan B, the 1,600-calorie-a-day plan, which is closest to her calorie intake of 1,500 for a weight loss.

If your calorie intake for weight loss is	Start with...
1,200 – 1,400	Plan A – 1,200 calories
1,500 – 1,800	Plan B – 1,600 calories
1,900 and over	Plan C – 2,000 calories

My initial daily meal plan will be Plan _____ with a _____ calories-per-day intake.

You may need to change your plan depending on your rate of weight loss. If you are losing less than one pound a week and you are on Plan B or C, you may want to switch to Plan A, increase your level of activity, or do both. If you are losing more than two pounds a week, you may want to switch to Plan B or C. Give the plan you are on at least one month before deciding to switch. Often the first few weeks of weight loss are more rapid than the following weeks. It may take this long for your body to settle into its normal rate of weight loss.

Step #9—Tracking Your Weight Loss

Select a time each week for weighing yourself to assess your rate of weight loss and make any adjustments necessary to your food or activity plans. In a notebook or on a piece of paper, track your weekly progress under the following headings:

Starting weight _____		Date _____
10 percent goal _____		BMI goal _____
Week #	**Present Weight**	**Pounds Lost**

Step #10—The Daily Meal Plans Serving List

Finally, it is time to look at the Daily Meal Plans Servings List. You will see that the servings list follows the same food groups of the nutrition pyramid that you were introduced to in Chapter 1. In the nutrition pyramid you were given a range of servings for each food group. In columns two, three, and four of the servings list that follows, you are given the exact number of daily servings per food group for each calorie plan. In the fifth column, to the right, you will see examples of serving sizes for these food groups. Once you have familiarized yourself with these serving sizes, you easily will be able to keep track of your food consumption.

The sixth column lists the number of calories per serving for that food group, which is very useful to know if you are using some of your pleasure food calories for extra servings of the basic food groups. In the last column, you will find examples of each food group. We will go into this in greater detail in Chapter 9 when you begin the actual meal plans. You might find it valuable to copy this page and keep it with you to consult throughout the day.

In this chapter, you have done a great deal of planning for getting started on the program. You now have all the basic tools you need to begin using the Daily Meal Plans for weight loss.

Figuring out the number of calories you need for weight maintenance and weight loss enabled you to determine your basic calorie requirements. By estimating how long it will take you to lose your desired amount of weight in a healthy way, you set up a realistic expectation for your progress, which, in turn, will help you avoid the discouragement that comes with impatience. In this chapter you were introduced to the servings list, the next chapter will give you the meal plans for the first three weeks of the program. This information will make it easier for you to make adjustments to the meal plans according to your own needs and lifestyle, when you eat out at restaurants, and when you begin to prepare your own meal plans from week four on.

The Daily Meal Plans Servings List

Food Groups	1,200 calories Plan A	1,600 calories Plan B	2,000 calories Plan C	Serving Sizes	Calories	Examples
Pleasure	180	240	300			wine, butter, sugar, chocolate
Low-fat/ Nonfat Dairy	2	3	3	8 oz. milk 1 cup yogurt 1-1/2 oz cheese	90	low/nonfat milk low/nonfat yogurt low/nonfat cheese
Lean Meat/ Beans	3	5	5½	1 oz meat 1/2 cup beans	55	lean, fat-trimmed meat, fish, skinless poultry, black beans, lentils
Nuts or Seeds	1	2	2	2 T	100	almonds, walnuts, sunflower seeds, sesame seeds
Plant Oils	3	4	5	1 tsp 1 T 2 T	45	vegetable oil (olive, canola, sunflower), low-fat mayonnaise, light salad dressing
Vegetables	3 or more	4 or more	5 or more	1/2 cup cooked, 1 cup raw leafy, 6 oz vegetable juice	25	broccoli, carrots, green beans, lettuce, tomatoes, squash, sweet potatoes
Fruits	2	3	4	1 medium fruit, 1/2 cup sliced fruit, 1/4 cup dried fruit	60	apricots, bananas, dates, oranges, grapefruit, berries, raisins, prunes
Whole Grains	4	5	6	1 slice bread, 1 oz dry cereal, 1/2 cup cooked rice, pasta or hot cereal	80	whole wheat bread, brown rice, whole wheat pasta, polenta, oatmeal

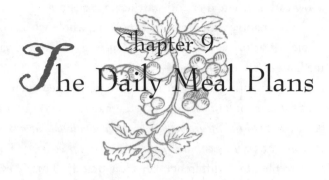

Chapter 9
The Daily Meal Plans

*One cannot think well, love well, sleep
well, if one has not dined well.*
—*Virginia Woolf*

In the California Wine Country Diet, you will be dining very well, indeed, as you enjoy delicious food that satisfies your nutritional needs and helps you to lose weight. But depending on your present diet, you will no doubt face some challenges as you begin following the California Wine Country Diet Meal Plans. We all enjoy our favorite treats and resist changing them. Let us look at some ways that you can continue eating the things you most love while opening up to new experiences. The basics of the California wine country nutrition pyramid come into play here.

Enjoying Whole Grains

Switching to whole grains will probably be one of the easiest changes you will need to make because almost all of the refined white-flour products you have enjoyed are also made in whole-grain versions: bread, cereals, tortillas, English muffins, waffles, pizza crust. Here are some tips for making the easy switch from refined white flour to whole grains:

• Get to know your local bakeries and try different whole-grain breads. Many bakeries will be happy to provide you a sample, if you ask.

- Pull out that bread machine that you put away when you went on a low-carbohydrate diet and start using it again.
- Stock your pantry with brown rice, polenta, whole-wheat couscous, whole-wheat pasta, and oatmeal. That way, you will always have the basis of a meal at hand.
- Experiment with grains you may have never tried such as buckwheat groats, bulgur, barley, millet, amaranth, and quinoa.
- *Be sure to read the nutrition labels of the whole-wheat products you purchase carefully. Look at the calories and fat content.* There can be a tremendous difference between brands. This is especially important with items you are going to be eating on a frequent basis such as tortillas. I recently saw two different whole-wheat tortilla brands both advertising their product as "low-carbohydrate." One brand had 80 calories per tortilla and the other 200 calories. The first would count as one grain serving, the second as two.

Enjoying Fruits

Fruits are the most refreshing, healthy, filling, and easy snacks you can find. Notice what fruit is in season and be sure to have some on hand.

- Keep a bowl of fresh fruit on the counter or even on your desk at work for everyone to enjoy. If the fruit is out where it can be seen, you will be more likely to pick up a piece and enjoy it.
- Grab a piece of fruit when you leave the house so you won't have to worry about being hungry later on.
- Look for recipes based on fruit (such as the ones in Chapter 10) to take the place of your refined sugar desserts.
- Keep a variety of dried fruit on hand to add to your cereal, salads, and as a back-up for when you have run out of fresh fruit. Keep in mind that ¼ cup of dried fruit equals one fruit serving.
- Keep bottles of lemon and lime juice available.
- Keep a variety of frozen unsweetened fruits, such as blueberries and strawberries, on hand to put on your cereal or in a smoothie.

- If you are going to drink fruit juice, choose a variety that is 100 percent juice, and remember that the serving size is ½ cup. You can also add a little fruit juice to sparkling water for flavor.
- To sweeten your yogurt or to top your toast in the morning look for 100 percent all-fruit spreads such as apple butter. Be sure to look at the number of calories per serving. If there are 20 or fewer calories per serving it can be counted as a free food. If there are more, use your pleasure food calories.

Enjoying Vegetables

If you do not already love vegetables, learn to. Supermarkets and farmers' markets offer a plethora of different, and even exotic, vegetables. Try them, because this is the one food group you can eat to your heart's content.

- When you visit a farmers' market and your local store, look for the best local, seasonal, and, if possible, organic produce.
- Salads and stir-fried vegetables are the best ways to fill your plate with nutritious food and minimal calories and minimal fat. Experiment with fat-free salad dressings such as the one included in the everyday recipes in Chapter 10. Add delicious flavor to a stir-fry with any of the many flavored sauces and shaker spice mixes that are available at your local supermarket. Make sure all condiments are low calorie.
- For a low-calorie/low-fat vegetable serving that you can easily keep on hand, make extra servings of the everyday vegetable soups from recipes in Chapter 10 and refrigerate or freeze them for later use.
- Keep vegetables such as peas, carrots, celery, and string beans ready as snacks.
- Keep frozen vegetables as back-ups for when fresh vegetables are out of season or when you have not gone to the store.
- Keep canned tomatoes, artichoke hearts, olives, and palm hearts in the cupboard.
- Vegetable juices such as tomato or carrot make quick and nutritious snacks or beverages to have with meals.

• Choose deep-colored vegetables such as yams, Swiss chard, carrots, and red peppers for added nutrition.

Enjoying Plant Oils

If you are used to cooking with lots of olive oil and pouring dressing all over your salad, you might find yourself having to make an adjustment to meet the plant-oil serving limits of this program. Try cutting back slowly, especially on creamy salad dressings, until your taste buds adjust. You will be surprised how quickly they do.

• To use a minimum of oil when frying, use a cooking spray. A one-second spritz covers a ten-inch skillet. When broiling or grilling vegetables or meat, spray the oil directly on the food. Buy one or more Misto oil sprayers. This sprayer requires slightly more work than the commercial spray cans because you have to pump it to pressurize it. The advantage is that you can fill the Misto with your favorite oil, and there are no chemicals or propellants. Find a store near you that sells these sprayers or visit www.misto.com online. A one-second spray of Misto equals ¼ teaspoon of oil, not enough to count as part of your daily oil serving.

• When dressing your salad at home, use one teaspoon of oil per person and toss your lettuce first, before adding lemon juice or vinegar and before putting in other vegetables. This will ensure that you are using the minimum amount of oil to cover the lettuce.

• When using a commercial dressing, find the one that you like best that has the lowest fat content, measure out a tablespoon, toss your salad, and then add one or two tablespoons of lemon juice.

• In restaurants, always ask for your dressing on the side. Dip your fork into the dressing and then into your salad. You can also use fresh lemon to make your dressing go farther.

• If you need more plant-oil servings for special dishes or when eating out, you can use your pleasure food calories (45 calories for 1 teaspoon of plant oil) or use one of your nut servings (1 tablespoon of nuts equals 1 teaspoon of plant oil).

• Experiment with different oils such as sesame, hazelnut, and walnut oils.

Enjoying Nuts or Seeds

Here is another nutritious food group that makes for a delicious and easy snack—and a healthy one when consumed in moderation.

• Keep a variety of raw and roasted, unsalted nuts and seeds on hand for putting on cereals, baking, and eating as a snack. See Chapter 1 for a list of recommended nuts and seeds.
• Do not eat nuts right out of the jar or package because you are likely to eat too many. Keep a tablespoon near your nuts and seeds so that you can easily measure out your servings.

Enjoying Lean Meat, Fish, Eggs, and Legumes

For most people, especially those who have been on high-protein diets, the servings of this group will seem very limited at first. Keep an open mind as you learn to eat in the pattern of healthy traditional diets, where protein is an accompaniment on the plate, rather than the focus of the meal.

• As suggested earlier in this book, have your meat or fish as part of another dish such as a salad, stir-fry, or burrito.
• As you are adjusting to the smaller-than-usual protein serving sizes, you may want to use some of your pleasure food calories for lean protein. One ounce of lean meat is 55 calories.
• You may also exchange a dairy serving (since it is also protein) for a lean meat serving, provided you have made up for the 500 mg of calcium through a supplement or other food.

Enjoying Low-fat/Nonfat Dairy

There are many ways to enjoy your low-fat or nonfat dairy servings.

• Nonfat or low-fat yogurt makes a wonderful breakfast, snack, or dessert, depending on what you mix with it: fruit, nuts, granola or all-fruit spreads. If you prefer to sweeten with regular sugar, count 15 pleasure food calories per teaspoon.

- Find your favorite brand of plain yogurt rather than yogurt with fruit mixed in. Read the label and select a nonfat or low-fat yogurt that has fewer than 110 calories per 8-ounce cup. If you select a brand with more than 110 calories, add the extra calories to your pleasure food calories for the day.

- One of the easiest ways to drink your dairy servings is in coffee or tea. So, put away that powdered creamer and half and half. Nonfat and low-fat dairy make for an excellent latté, cappuccino, or chai tea that you can make at home or buy at your favorite coffee shop. You can sweeten these drinks with either a sugar substitute or real sugar (using 15 pleasure food calories per teaspoon). If you are at home, you may want to add two tablespoons of light whipped topping for no extra calories.

- Instead of the half and half or cream called for in recipes, use evaporated skim milk.

- Make your own fat-free cream cheese by setting plain fat-free yogurt in cheese cloth over a bowl for a few hours.

Enjoying Cheese

Cheese is an integral part of the California Wine Country Diet, whether it's goat cheese on a salad or fresh feta in a pita pocket, cheese adds its unique signature, while bringing the flavors together in a dish. Like milk or yogurt, cheese is a good source of calcium. However, most natural cheeses are made from whole milk and cream, which contribute saturated fat and extra calories to your diet. In the Daily Meal Plan Serving List, you will note that for most low-fat cheeses, 1½ ounces is considered one dairy serving.

Limit your dairy from whole-milk cheeses to no more than one-half of your daily dairy servings. The remainder should come from nonfat or low-fat dairy foods such as nonfat/low-fat milk and yogurt. This way you will be able to enjoy cheese while still keeping your saturated fat and calorie intake in check. If you wish to have more whole-milk cheese servings in a day, you will need to use your pleasure food calories.

Nonfat/low-fat Cheese	Serving Size	Calories
(<6.0 gms fat/serving)		
Cottage cheese, 1% fat	½ cup	82.0
"Diet cheese" (<55 calories/oz)	1½ ounces	82.5
Feta	1½ ounces	75.0
Goat (Chevre)	1 ounce	76.0
Laughing Cow, light	2 wedges	70.0
Mozzarella, part-skim	1½ ounces	72.0
Parmesan, grated	¼ cup	92.0
Ricotta, part-skim	¼ cup	86.0

Medium-fat Cheese
(6.1 - 8.0 gms fat/serving)

Brie	1 ounce	100.0
Camembert	1 ounce	85.0
Gouda	1 ounce	101.0
Gorgonzola	1 ounce	93.0
Mozzarella, whole-milk	1 ounce	80.0
Provolone	1 ounce	100.0
Swiss	1 ounce	107.0

High-fat Cheese
(8.1+ gms fat/serving)

Blue	1 ounce	100.0
Cheddar	1 ounce	114.0
Colby	1 ounce	112.0
Gruyere	1 ounce	117.0
Havarti	1 ounce	121.0
Monterey Jack	1 ounce	106.0
Muenster	1 ounce	104.0

Since cheeses vary in the amount of fat and calories they have per ounce, you cannot always count on the 1½-ounce rule. The list on the previous page will guide you in choosing the appropriate amount of cheese that can be considered one dairy serving. Dairy foods that have little to no calcium, such as cream cheese, cream, and butter, are not part of the group. The calories for each serving are also listed in case you will be using pleasure food calories for your cheese.

Enjoying Pleasure Foods

Happily, you will start selecting—and enjoying—pleasure foods in your diet from the first day of this program. Remember, with this program there is no need to deny yourself. There is only the need to remain conscious of your choices.

One area of particular challenge within the pleasure food category is how best to enjoy sugar and other sweeteners. I still remember my son's introduction to sugar at about the age of three. It was love at first bite! We human beings naturally enjoy sweetness. We crave it.

While our ancestors usually got their sugar in the form of fruit, today sugar is found everywhere we look—not only in sodas and donuts, but in a wide variety of processed foods from ketchup to cereal. It is estimated that the average American consumes 150 pounds of sugar a year.

Sugar is the subject of major controversy in the field of nutrition and has been accused of causing many health problems including obesity, insulin resistance, hyperactivity, and tooth decay.

The California Wine Country Diet recommends that you try to enjoy sweetness, first of all, from the natural taste of fresh foods. As mentioned, replace sugar-laden jams with lower calorie spreads made from 100 percent fruit. When you do consume foods or beverages with added sweeteners, do so with conscious indulgence.

Always measure the amount of the added sweetener, and count it as part of your daily pleasure food calories. Natural sweeteners you may want to add to your food include sugar, honey, maple syrup, and rice syrup. They are all in the range of 40 to 60 calories per tablespoon. While you may prefer a particular sweetener, to your body they are all equivalent to sugar. Save your sweetener calories for those times and foods when you will most enjoy them. One very simple way to reduce calories and still enjoy sweets is to lower the level of sweetness. If you are used to a tablespoon of sugar in your coffee, try slowly cutting that amount to one teaspoon, and you will save 30 calories per cup.

Artificial sweeteners have been a mainstay of dieting Americans. The truckloads of diet sodas and other products sweetened with artificial sweeteners have certainly not solved the continuing weight problems of our population. Moreover, there is considerable concern over the health risks associated with these products. If you decide to use an artificial sweetener, at this point the safest one appears to be sucralose which is sold under the brand name Splenda. It is made through a multistep process that starts with sugar and selectively replaces three hydrogen-oxygen groups on the sugar molecule with three chlorine atoms. Since it is a chemically altered food, to be on the safe side it is recommended for only limited use.

Natural sweeteners which can add sweetness with fewer or no calories include Xylitol and Stevia. Xylitol was first manufactured by a German chemist in 1891. A natural substance found in fibrous vegetables and fruit, it is used in a number of countries including Germany and Japan as the preferred sweetener in diabetic diets. Xylitol has 40 percent fewer calories and 75 percent fewer carbohydrates than sugar. It has been found to benefit oral health and is being studied for other health benefits. When first used, it can cause mild diarrhea or cramping in some people.

Stevia is a South American shrub whose leaves have been used for centuries to sweeten beverages. It is virtually calorie free and many times sweeter than sugar. Stevia has not been approved by the FDA for use in foods but can be bought in health food stores as a dietary supplement. There are health concerns about use of Stevia in large amounts, which is why it has not been approved as a food additive. Used one or two times a day to sweeten a beverage, as has been done by native people in Paraguay and Brazil for centuries, it does not appear to pose a health threat.

Chapter 11 is devoted to wine and other pleasure foods, so you might want to look ahead and review the discussion there before beginning the Daily Meal Plans.

Here are some ideas to help you in dealing with pleasure foods:

- Make a list of your favorite pleasure foods with their calories and serving sizes. (Use a calorie-counting book or the list in Chapter 11.)
- Be sure to keep track of your pleasure food calories.
- Be sure to use up all your pleasure food calories so that your calorie level does not get too low.
- Enjoy these calories, and make sure to always consult your fun-loving basic self about what it wants.

Enjoying Free Foods

Yes, there are foods that you can eat without worrying about where they fit into the program. Here is the rule: Generally, foods and beverages that contain 20 or fewer calories a serving are allowable without worrying about the calories. When *no* serving size is specified, you can eat or drink as much of the item as you wish. For those items listed with specific serving sizes, you can eat two or three servings a day.

Beverages
Bouillon or broth without fat
Bouillon, low sodium
Carbonated water
Club soda
(can be high in sodium; look for sodas with no salt added)
Coffee
Tea
Cocoa powder, unsweetened (1 tablespoon)

Condiments
Apple butter (1 tablespoon)
Ketchup (1 tablespoon)
Flavored vinegars
100 percent all-fruit spreads
(2 teaspoons, or no more than 20 calories)
Horseradish sauce
Mustard

Pickles, dill, non-sweetened
Salad dressing, fat-free (2 tablespoons)
Salsa (¼ cup)

Dairy
Cream cheese, fat free (1 tablespoon)
Mayonnaise, fat free (1 tablespoon)
Sour cream, fat free (1 tablespoon)
Whipped topping, regular or light (2 tablespoons)

Fruit
Cranberries, unsweetened (½ cup)
Rhubarb, unsweetened (½ cup)

Pan Spray
All commercial pan sprays
Your favorite oil from a Misto sprayer

Raw Vegetables (1 cup)
Cabbage
Celery
Chinese cabbage
Cucumber
Green onion
Hot peppers
Mushrooms
Radishes
Zucchini

Salad Greens
Endive
Escarole
Lettuce
Spinach

Seasonings

Basil

Celery seed

Cinnamon

Chili powder

Chives

Curry

Dill

Flavoring extracts (almond, vanilla, walnut, or others)

Garlic and garlic powder

Herbs and spices that contain no added sugar

Lemon and lime juice for flavor

Mint

Onion powder

Oregano

Paprika

Pepper

Pimiento

Salt

Soy sauce and low-sodium soy sauce

Wine, for cooking (¼ cup)

Worcestershire sauce

Sweet Substitutes

Gum, sugar-free

Xylitol

Stevia

Enjoying All Aspects of the Wheel of Weight-Management

The California Wine Country Diet Meal Plans were created to include all the different aspects of the Wheel of Weight-Management. By following the meal plans for your calorie level, you will meet all your daily nutritional requirements. You will be establishing a nutritional pattern that will lead to lifelong good-health habits. The Daily

Meal Plans will provide you the opportunity to increase physical activity. If you have been eating frequently at restaurants, driving through fast food take-out lines, or zapping frozen dinners, your level of daily activity will certainly go up as you search stores, walk through the farmers' market, and prepare your own food at home.

The California Wine Country Diet strikes a balance between practicality, pleasure, and variety. While it is impossible to devise a plan that exactly meets everyone's lifestyle, the Daily Meal Plans are practical for most people. Though you can start on any day, the meal plans assume you will begin on a Monday.

Breakfasts introduce you to a variety of meal ideas while requiring minimal preparation. Lunches are also designed with minimal preparation in mind. Many lunches include leftovers from a previous day's dinner. All are dishes that are easy to bring with you to work or to otherwise eat on the run. Three nights a week you will have dinners from the Everyday Menu, which contains meals designed to be simple to prepare and that allow you to learn basic recipes and then experiment and create variety from those basics. Four nights a week you will have dinners from recipes by some of the finest chefs at California wine country restaurants. Once you have followed your meal plans for three full weeks, you can begin to incorporate into your diet the additional enticing restaurant recipes. (See Chapter 12.) As you experiment with new foods and new ways of preparation, you will, of course, find that you like some dishes better than others. When you are at the place in this program where you can create your own food plans, go ahead and enjoy these recipes as often as you wish.

Most of the evening meals are those that will please people of all ages, so you can share them with your household. The dinners on days four, five, six, and seven may require somewhat more preparation, but they make great meals for entertaining. No longer will family and friends avoid eating with you because "you're on a diet." Soon they'll be begging for an invitation to dinner.

The meal plans are designed not only to help you lose weight and enhance your health, they are also designed to educate you. By the end of the first three weeks on your plan, you should feel confident about creating your own meal plans and will know what portion sizes you should be eating. Here are some additional tools to help you make the most of the Daily Meal Plans.

Meal Plan Tool #1 —
The Daily Meal Plans Serving List

Make at least two copies of the Daily Meal Plans Serving List. (See page 158, Chapter 8.) One is for home and one is to take with you. The serving list tells you exactly how many daily servings you should have for each food group and lists examples of these foods. After using the Daily Meal Plans Servings List for a while, it will become second nature to you and will make meal planning easy.

Meal Plan Tool #2 —
Measurement Equivalents by Capacity

Dash = less than 1/8 teaspoon

3 teaspoons = 1 tablespoon

2 tablespoons = 1 fluid ounce

4 tablespoons = ¼ cup

8 tablespoons = ½ cup

12 tablespoons = ¾ cup

16 tablespoons = 1 cup

8 ounces = 1 cup

1 cup = ½ pint

2 cups = 1 pint

2 pints (4 cups) = 1 quart

4 quarts (liquid) = 1 gallon

Measurement Equivalents by Weight

1 ounce = 28.35 grams

3.57 ounces = 100 grams

16 ounces = 1 pound

Meal Plan Tool #3 —
Portion Estimation

When you are in a situation where you cannot weigh and measure your portions, here are some visual comparisons to help you estimate:

1 medium apple or peach = the size of a tennis ball

1 ounce of cheese = the size of 4 stacked dice

1 cup of mashed potatoes or broccoli = the size of a man's fist

3 ounces of meat = the size and thickness of a deck of playing cards

1 teaspoon of oil or butter = about the size of the tip of your thumb

2 tablespoons of nuts = (covers) the palm of a small hand.

Meal Plan Tool #4 —
The Daily Meal Plan Form

The Daily Meal Plan form on the following page is designed to help you learn how to plan your meals and to assist you in keeping track of what you are eating. You can copy this form or download it from www.CaliforniaWineCountryDiet.com. Even though you will be given meal plans for the first three weeks, it is a good idea to start using the form from Day #1. You will then have a record of exactly what you ate, and it can also give you ideas for planning your own meals later on. Keeping food records has been found to correlate highly with successful weight loss and weight maintenance. The Daily Meal Plan form makes keeping such records easy.

At the top of the form, you will see the servings for each calorie level. As you go through your day, mark off the corresponding box after you have eaten a serving. Below the serving list, you have space to write what you actually did eat at each meal, for your snacks, and pleasure foods. You can also use this form to record your opinions on the different recipes as you try them and later to create menu plans.

Finally, at the bottom of the Daily Meal Plan form you will see the "5-Star Rating" system. This is your chance to rate yourself on how you did on all the different aspects of the Wheel of Weight-Management. Give yourself a rating from 1 to 5, depending on how you did overall on each aspect that day. The 5-Star Rating system recognizes the fullness of your life and reminds you to appreciate yourself for all that you are doing.

The California Wine Country Diet Daily Meal Plan Form

	Plan A					Plan B						Plan C					
Pleasure Foods	180 calories ❑					240 calories ❑						300 calories ❑					
Low/Nonfat Dairy	2 servings ❑❑					3 servings ❑❑❑						3 servings ❑❑❑					
Lean Meat/Beans	3 servings ❑❑❑					5 servings ❑❑❑❑❑						5.5 servings ❑❑❑❑❑❑					
Nuts or Seeds	1 servings ❑					2 servings ❑❑						2 servings ❑❑					
Plant Oils	3 servings ❑❑❑					4 servings ❑❑❑❑						5 servings ❑❑❑❑❑					
Vegetables	3+ servings ❑❑❑❑					4+ servings ❑❑❑❑❑						5+ servings ❑❑❑❑❑					
Fruits	2 servings ❑❑					3 servings ❑❑❑						4 servings ❑❑❑❑					
Whole Grains	4 servings ❑❑❑❑					5 servings ❑❑❑❑❑						6 servings ❑❑❑❑❑❑					

Meal #1   Breakfast

Today's date:

Meal #2   Morning Snack

Meal #3   Lunch

Meal #4   Afternoon Snack

Meal #5   Dinner

Pleasure Foods   (Plan A =180 Calories, Plan B =240 Calories, Plan C = 300 Calories)

5 Star Rating — Rate how you feel you did overall today in regard to each aspect of the Wheel of Weight-Management, from 1 (the lowest) to 5 (the highest):

Nutrition _____   Physical Activity _____   Practicality _____
Pleasure _____   Relationships _____   Variety _____

Photocopy this form or download it from www.CaliforniaWineCountryDiet.com.

Meal Plan Tool #5 —
21 Days of Daily Meal Plans

You are now ready to start the daily meals plans. The first three days are called "Simple Start," because the meals require minimal preparation. During these three Simple Start days, I suggest that you do not drink alcohol. Instead, you can use your pleasure food calories for added servings of the basic food groups or for your other favorite foods as you adjust to what may be a new way of eating.

Following each serving item you will be given in parentheses the nutritional exchange for that food. This exchange information will enable you to easily make changes in the meal plan. For example, if you are on Plan A, then on Day #1 the meal plan for breakfast says "Oatmeal—½ cup (1 grain)." If you dislike oatmeal, you will see that you can exchange it for one grain serving. You look at the serving list and decide to have a piece of toast instead of oatmeal. You would then check off one grain on your Daily Meal Plan form. The exchanges also can help you make good decisions when you eat out. On Plan A, if you were going out to dinner on Day #1, you would look for a selection at the restaurant menu that has approximately 2.5 protein, 2 vegetables, 3 oil, and 2 grain servings. You might order fish with a salad and rice. Since it can be difficult to estimate restaurant servings and ingredients, you can use some of your pleasure food calories as a safety net and bring home leftovers, because restaurant serving sizes tend to be large.

Different ways to follow the meal plans include

- Follow them exactly as they are written.
- Exchange individual food items for another serving from the serving list.
- Use a food serving at a different time of the day.
- Exchange an entire meal or meals for equivalent servings. Make sure to keep track of the servings you are using on the Daily Meal Plan form. Starting in Week Two you will be given some meals and snacks to create on your own, using the specified nutritional servings. This will give you practice in creating your own meal plans.

Week Four and Beyond

The California Wine Country Diet is not a diet with phases but rather one that establishes lifelong eating patterns. The Epilogue, Forever After, will explore the issues of weight plateaus and weight maintenance.

If you have lost all the weight you need to lose by the end of twenty-one days, go to the recommendations in the Epilogue for weight maintenance. If you have more weight to lose, there are a variety of ways to continue on the program:

- The simplest way is to begin again at Day #1 and follow the Daily Meals Plans as given.
- You might want to continue following the given Daily Meals Plans making substitutions from the serving list for individual food items.
- You could vary the days of the meal plans to have the ones you most enjoy. Your nutritional needs are met within each individual day. If you do vary the order of the days, you will need to plan for meals that make use of leftovers from the previous days.
- You may feel ready to begin creating your own Daily Meal Plans based on the food group servings for your calorie plan. You can use the Daily Meal Plan form to create menus and to check off the serving boxes to make sure that you are getting all your daily servings.

It is important that you begin creating your own Daily Meal Plans either at some point during weight loss or immediately upon moving into weight maintenance. That way you will be prepared to be on your own and will not fall into old eating patterns just because you are "off the diet."

One simple way that I have found to create my own meal plans is to establish a consistent daily pattern. For example, you might always have a grain, a fruit, and a dairy serving at breakfast. Your morning snack might always be nuts, and your afternoon snack might always be fruit. That leaves lunch and dinner to think about. Depending on what is going on in your life, you may decide to have all your protein at one of those meals or divide your protein servings between both meals. While the first three weeks are designed to introduce you to a wide variety of foods and patterns of eating, when you have seen what works for you, having a regular pattern, especially during the work week, can make life easier. Save variety and exciting new foods for the evenings and weekends.

At last, you are ready to start Day #1 of the California Wine Country Diet Daily Meal Plans. Here is a shopping list for the first three Simple Start days to help you get off to an easy beginning. Many of the items on the list you may already have. Most will be used again in future meals. Now enjoy yourself!

Simple-Start Shopping List

Bread
Whole-wheat bread
Whole-wheat English muffins
Whole-wheat hamburger buns
Whole-wheat pita bread
Whole-wheat tortillas (80 calories or less)

Condiments—herbs, spices
Apple butter
Chili powder
Cumin
100 percent all-fruit spread (20 calories or less per 2-teaspoon serving)
Ketchup
Mustard, grainy
Olive oil, extra virgin
Oregano, fresh or dried
Pepper, ground black
Pickles, dill
Rosemary—fresh
Salt—kosher

Dairy
Cheddar cheese, low-fat (less than 55 calories per ounce)

Cottage cheese, nonfat/low-fat

Eggs

Feta cheese, solid or crumbled

Milk, nonfat or 1 percent

Mozzarella cheese, part-skim

Orange juice

Sour cream, fat-free

Yogurt, nonfat/low-fat (110 calories per cup or less)

Meat

Chicken breast, bone in or out (1 per person with enough left over
for Day #2)

Ground meat—beef or turkey or vegetarian patty—your choice

Nuts

Almonds

Pistachios

Walnuts, shelled and in pieces

Package

Artichoke hearts—in water

Black beans, 15-oz can or package of dried beans

Brown rice

Coffee

Hummus—1 can garbanzo beans and sesame tahini if making
hummus recipe (or package of dried hummus or prepared hummus
at deli counter)

Oatmeal, regular

Olives (optional)—black Greek kalamata

Tea—green tea highly recommended

V-8 or tomato juice—low sodium

Produce

Alfalfa sprouts

Avocado

Blueberries, fresh or frozen
Carrots
Celery
Cilantro
Cucumber
Garlic, fresh cloves
Green beans
Lemons or lemon juice
Lettuce, romaine
Onions, red (2)
Oranges
Parsley, Italian
Red bell peppers (optional—yellow, orange or green also)
Spinach
Strawberries, fresh or frozen
Tangerines
Tomatoes, several

Free—Review the free foods listed earlier in this chapter for other items you might like to have on hand.

California Wine Country Diet Meal Plans

Here now are the Meal Plans for the first three weeks.

Daily Meal Plan: Day #1 — Simple Start

To substitute a food item, refer to the Daily Meal Plans Servings List on page 158.

Meal #1
Breakfast—Oatmeal with Walnuts and Strawberries

Food	Plan	Serving
Oatmeal with cinnamon	A & B	½ cup cooked .. (1 grain)
	C	1 cup cooked ... (2 grains)
made or served with —		
nonfat/low-fat milk	A	½ cup .... (.5 dairy)
	B & C	1 cup .... (1 dairy)
Sliced strawberries	A	½ cup .... (1 fruit)
	B	1 cup .... (2 fruit)
	C	1½ cups .... (3 fruit)
Walnuts in small pieces	A	2 T .... (1 nut)
	B & C	4 T .... (2 nuts)
Coffee or tea with		
nonfat/low-fat milk	A B & C	½ cup milk ...... (.5 dairy)

Meal #2
Morning Snack—Yogurt

Food	Plan	Serving
Nonfat/low-fat plain yogurt	A B & C	½ cup .... (.5 dairy)
100% fruit spread	A B & C	2 tsp .... (free)

Meal #3
Lunch—Hummus and Vegetable Pita Sandwich

Food	Plan	Serving
Whole-wheat pita bread	A	½ piece .... (1 grain)
	B & C	1 whole piece .. (2 grains)

Hummus	A	¼ cup	(.5 protein)
	B & C	½ cup	(1 protein)

(See recipe in Chapter 10 or use store-bought hummus.)

Lettuce, tomato, sprouts,	A	1 cup	(1 vegetable)
	B & C	2 cups	(2 vegetable)

(Add red peppers, lemon juice, salt/pepper to taste.)

Feta cheese	A	¾ oz	(.5 dairy)
	B & C	1½ oz	(1 dairy)

Meal #4
Afternoon Snack—Orange

Food	Plan	Serving
Orange	A B & C	1 medium .... (1 fruit)

Meal #5
Dinner—Broiled Chicken with Rice and Green Beans

Food	Plan	Serving
Broiled chicken breast	A	2½ oz	(2.5 protein)
	B	4.0 oz	(4 protein)
	C	4½ oz	(4.5 protein)

(Spray with olive oil; season with minced garlic, rosemary, salt, and pepper. Remove skin before eating. Save leftover chicken for tomorrow's lunch.)

Green string beans	A & B	1 cup	(2 vegetable)
	C	1½ cups	(3 vegetable)

A la Chef John Ash: "Put green beans in slightly salted boiling water for 3 minutes, take them out, drain. Drizzle with good quality olive oil; season with a little salt and pepper."

Olive oil	A	3 tsp	(3 oil)
	B	4 tsp	(4 oil)
	C	5 tsp	(5 oil)
Brown rice	A B & C	1 cup	(2 grains)

Today's pleasure foods	A	180 calories	
	B	240 calories	
	C	300 calories	

Recommendation: No alcoholic beverages for the first three days.

Meal #1
Breakfast—Egg with Toast

Food	Plan	Serving	
Egg—poached or boiled	A B & C	1 egg	(1 protein)
Whole-wheat toast	A & B	1 slice	(1 grain)
	C	2 slices	(2 grain)
Apple butter on toast	A B & C	1 T	(free)
Coffee or tea with nonfat/low-fat milk	A B & C	½ cup milk	(.5 dairy)

Meal #2
Morning Snack—Almonds and Tangerine

Food	Plan	Serving	
Almonds	A	2 T	(1 nut)
	B & C	4 T	(2 nut)
Tangerine	A & B	1	(1 fruit)
	C	2	(2 fruit)

Meal #3
Lunch—Greek Salad with Chicken
(See recipe in Chapter 10.)

Food	Plan	Serving	
Greek Salad	A & B	2 cups salad	(2 vegetable)
	C	3 cups salad	(3 vegetable)
Lemon and olive oil dressing	A & B	1 T	(2 oil)
	C	1½ T	(3 oil)
Cubed broiled chicken	A	1 oz	(1 protein)
	B	2 oz	(2 protein)
	C	2½ oz	(2.5 protein)
Feta cheese	A	¾ oz	(.5 dairy)
	B & C	1½ oz	(1 dairy)

| Whole-wheat pita bread | A B & C | 1 whole piece .. (2 grains) |
| Kalamata olives (optional) | A B & C | 5 olives .... 45 pleasure food calories |

Meal #4

Afternoon Snack—Yogurt and Blueberries

Food	Plan	Serving
Plain nonfat/low-fat yogurt	A	1 cup .... (1 dairy)
	B & C	1½ cup .... (1.5 dairy)
Blueberries, fresh or frozen	A	½ cup .... (1 fruit)
	B & C	1 cup .... (2 fruit)

Note: Use calorie-free sweetener in yogurt if desired.

Meal #5

Dinner—Black Bean Burritos

(See recipe in Chapter 10.)

Food	Plan	Serving
Black bean burritos	A	1½ cup filling . (1 oil, 2 vegetable, 1 protein)
	B & C	3 cups filling ... (2 oil, 4 vegetable, 2 protein)
Whole-wheat tortillas	A	1 .... (1 grain)
	B & C	2 .... (2 grain)
(80 calories or less per tortilla)		
Serve with fat-free sour creamand	A B & C	1 T .... (free)
fresh salsa	A B & C	¼ cup .... (free)
V-8 juice (low sodium)	A B & C	6 oz .... (1 vegetable)
Today's pleasure foods	A	180 calories
	B	240 calories
	C	300 calories

Recommendation: No alcoholic beverages for the first three days.

Daily Meal Plan: Day #3 — Simple Start

To substitute a food item, refer to the Daily Meal Plans Servings List on page 158.

Meal #1
Breakfast—Fruit Smoothie & English Muffin

Food	Plan	Serving
Fruit smoothie—Mix in a blender		
Nonfat/low-fat milk	A B & C	1 cup .... (1 dairy)
Blueberries, fresh or frozen	A	¼ cup .... (.5 fruit)
	B & C	½ cup .... (1 fruit)
Strawberries, fresh or frozen	A	¼ cup .... (.5 fruit)
	B & C	½ cup .... (1 fruit)
Orange juice	A & B	½ cup .... (1 fruit)
	C	1 cup .... (2 fruit)
Ice	A B & C	½ cup .... (free)
Protein powder (optional)	A B & C	Use pleasure food calories
English muffin	A	½ muffin .... (1 grain)
	B & C	1 muffin .... (2 grain)
Apple butter on muffin	A B & C	1 T .... (free)

Meal #2
Morning Snack—Pistachios

Food	Plan	Serving
Pistachios (shelled)	A	2 T .... (1 nut)
	B & C	4 T .... (2 nut)

Meal #3
Lunch—Avocado Wrap

Food	Plan	Serving
Avocado, sliced	A	¼ .... (2 oil)
	B	1/3 .... (3 oil)
	C	½ .... (4 oil)
Whole-wheat tortilla	A & B	1 .... (1 grain)
	C	2 .... (2 grain)

(80 calories or less per tortilla)

Tomato, medium size, sliced	A B & C .... 1 tomato .... (1 vegetable)
Lettuce and alfalfa sprouts	A B & C .... 1 cup .... (1 vegetable)
Low-fat cheddar cheese	A .... None
	B & C .... 1½ oz .... (1 dairy)

(55 calories or less per oz.)

| V-8 or tomato juice (low sodium) | A B & C .... 6 oz .... (1 vegetable) |

Meal #4

Afternoon Snack—Celery Filled with Cottage Cheese

Food	Plan	Serving
Celery	A B & C .... 3 or 4 stalks .... (1 vegetable)
Nonfat/low-fat cottage cheese	A B & C .... ½ cup .... (1 dairy)
Season to taste with salsa	A B & C .... ¼ cup .... (free)

Meal #5

Dinner—Burgers (turkey or beef or vegetarian)

Food	Plan	Serving
Ground lean patty	A .... 3 oz .... (3 protein)
	B .... 5 oz .... (5 protein)
	C .... 5½ oz .... (5.5 protein)

Season with salt, pepper, and minced garlic; cook with 1 teaspoon canola oil per patty.

| Whole-wheat hamburger bun | A B & C .... 1 whole bun ... (2 grains) |
| Lettuce, tomatoes garnish | A B & C .... 1 cup+ .... (1+ vegetable) |

Add the free foods pickles, ketchup, and mustard to taste.

Today's pleasure foods	A .... 180 calories
	B .... 240 calories
	C .... 300 calories

Recommendation: No alcoholic beverages for the first three days.

Meal #1

Breakfast—Waffles Topped with Strawberries and Yogurt

Food	Plan	Serving
Whole-wheat frozen waffles—toasted	A & B	1 waffle .... (1 grain)
	C	2 waffles .... (2 grain)
Plain nonfat/low-fat yogurt	A	½ cup .... (.5 dairy)
	B & C	1½ cups .... (1.5 dairy)
Strawberries —sliced	A	½ cup .... (1 fruit)
	B	1 cup .... (2 fruit)
	C	1½ cups .... (3 fruit)
Coffee or tea with nonfat/low-fat milk	A B & C	½ cup milk ..... (.5 dairy)

Meal #2

Morning Snack—Pear

Food	Plan	Serving
Pear	A B & C	1 pear .... (1 fruit)

Meal #3

Lunch—Turkey Sandwich

Food	Plan	Serving
Whole-wheat bread	A	slice .... (1 grain)
	B & C	2 slices .... (2 grain)
Turkey, deli sliced	A	3 oz .... (3 protein)
	B	5 oz .... (5 protein)
	C	5½ oz .... (5.5 protein)
Lettuce, tomato, sprouts, pickles, mustard	A	1 cup .... (1 vegetable)
	B & C	2 cups .... (2 vegetable)

Meal #4
Afternoon Snack—Popcorn

Food	Plan	Serving
Popcorn, popped, no fat added or low-fat microwave	A B & C .... 3 cups .... (1 grain)	

Meal #5
Dinner—Los Olivos Café Panzanella Salad
(See recipe in Chapter 12.)

Food	Plan	Serving
Café Panzanella salad	A B & C .... 2½ cups .... (2 vegetable, 1 grain)	
topped with Gorgonzola cheese	A B & C .... 1 oz .... (1 dairy)	
and crunched pistachios	A .... 2 T .... (1 nut)	
	B & C .... 4 T .... (2 nut)	
Salad Dressing	A .... 1 T .... (3 oil)	
	B .... 1½ T .... (4 oil)	
	C .... 2 T .... (5 oil)	
Today's pleasure foods	A .... 180 calories	
	B .... 240 calories	
	C .... 300 calories	

If you wish to have wine with dinner, Chef Nat Ely of the Los Olivos Café (which you may have seen in the movie Sideways*) recommends Sangiovese, Barbera, or Pinot Noir.*

Daily Meal Plan: Day #5
To substitute a food item, refer to the Daily Meal Plans Servings List on page 158.

Meal #1
Breakfast—Cereal

Food	Plan	Serving
Whole-grain cereal	A	1 oz .... (1 grain)
	B	2 oz .... (2 grain)
	C	3 oz .... (3 grain)
Nonfat/low-fat milk	A	½ cup .... (.5 dairy)
	B & C	1 cup .... (1 dairy)
Banana sliced on top	A	None
	B	½ cup .... (1 fruit)
	C	1 cup .... (2 fruit)
Coffee or tea with nonfat/low-fat milk	A B & C	½ cup milk ..... (.5 dairy)

Meal #2
Morning Snack—Orange

Food	Plan	Serving
Orange	A B & C	1 (1 fruit)

Meal #3
Lunch—Apple-Walnut Salad
(See recipe in Chapter 10.)

Food	Plan	Serving
Apple walnut salad	A B & C	1½ cups .... (1 fruit, 2 vegetable)
Red leaf lettuce	A B & C	1cup or more ... (1+ vegetable)
Chopped walnuts	A	2 T .... (1 nut)
	B & C	4 T .... (2 nut)
Gorgonzola cheese	A	1 oz................ (1 dairy)
	B & C	1½ oz .... (1.5 dairy)
Dressing	A B & C	½ cup .... (free)

Meal #4
Afternoon Snack—Cream Cheese, Crackers & Greek Olives

Food	Plan	Serving
Whole-wheat crackers	A B & C	5 crackers .... (1 grain)
with fat-free cream cheese	A B & C	1 to 2 T .... (free)
Black kalamata olives	A B & C	10 olives .... (2 oil)

Meal #5
Dinner—Benbow Inn Grilled Wild Salmon with Dill and Yogurt Mashed Potatoes and Whole Grained Mustard Vinaigrette
(See recipe in Chapter 12.)

Food	Plan	Serving
Benbow Inn grilled wild salmon	A	3 oz .... (3 protein)
	B	5 oz .... (5 protein)
	C	5½ oz .... (5.5 protein)

Cook extra salmon and save for Day #6 lunch.

Food	Plan	Serving
Dill and yogurt mashed potatoes	A B & C	1 cup .... (2 grain)
Vinaigrette	A	1½ T .... (1 oil)
	B	3 T .... (2 oil)
	C	4½ T .... (3 oil)

Save extra vinaigrette for Day #6 lunch.

Food	Plan	Serving
Asparagus—steamed and seasoned with lemon juice	A B & C	1+ cups .... (2+ vegetable)

	Plan	Serving
Today's pleasure foods	A	180 calories
	B	240 calories
	C	300 calories

If you wish to have wine with dinner, Chef Marci Bame suggests Sauvignon Blanc or Chardonnay. For more details see the recipe.

Meal #1

Breakfast—Scrambled Eggs, Bagel & Cream Cheese

Food	Plan	Serving
Whipped egg(s)	A	1 egg (1 protein)
	B & C	2 eggs (2 protein)
with nonfat/low-fat milk	A	¼ cup (.25 dairy)
	B & C	½ cup (.5 dairy)
Whole-grain bagel, toasted	A	½ bagel (1 grain)
	B & C	1 bagel (2 grain)
with fat-free cream cheese	A B &C	1 T (free)
100% fruit spread	A B & C	2 tsp (free)
Coffee or tea		
with nonfat/low-fat milk	A	¼ cup (.25 dairy)
	B & C	½ cup (.5 dairy)

Meal #2

Morning Snack—Yogurt with Raspberries & Granola

Food	Plan	Serving
Plain nonfat/low-fat yogurt	A	½ cup (.5 dairy)
	B & C	1 cup (1 dairy)
Raspberries, fresh or frozen	A	½ cup (1 fruit)
	B & C	1 cup (2 fruit)
Granola, low-fat	A B & C	¼ cup (1 grain)

Meal #3

Lunch—Cold Salmon Salad

Food	Plan	Serving
Cold salmon from		
Day #5 dinner	A	2 oz (2 protein)
	B	3 oz (3 protein)
	C	3½ oz (3.5 protein)
Salad of spring greens,		
cucumbers, tomatoes	A B & C	2+ cups (2+ vegetable)

Benbow Inn vinaigrette
from Day #5 dinner

A .... 1½ T .... (1 oil)
B .... 3 T .... (2 oil)
C .... 4½ T .... (3 oil)

Bread sticks

A & B .... 2 sticks .... (1 grain)
C .... 4 sticks .... (2 grain)

Meal #4

Afternoon Snack—Baked Apple and Walnuts
(See recipe in Chapter 10.)

Food   Plan   Serving

Baked apple

A & B .... 1 apple .... (1 fruit)
C .... 2 apples .... (2 fruit)

Walnuts—chopped

A .... 2 T .... (1 nut)
B & C .... 4 T .... (2 nut)

Meal #5

Dinner—Little River Inn Grilled Eggplant and Portabella Mushrooms with Tomato and Sweet Pepper Sauce
(See recipe in Chapter 12.)

Food   Plan   Serving

Little River Inn grilled
eggplant and portabella
mushrooms   A B & C .... ¼ of recipe ..... (1 dairy,
                                                 5 vegetable, 2 oil)

Italian bread, spray and grill   A B & C .... 1 slice .... (1 grain)

Today's pleasure foods

A .... 180 calories
B .... 240 calories
C .... 300 calories

If you wish to have wine with dinner, Chef Silver Canul suggests a Pinot Noir.

Meal #1

Breakfast—Oatmeal with Walnuts & Raisins

Food	Plan	Serving
Oatmeal with cinnamon	A & B	½ cup cooked . (1 grain)
	C	1 cup cooked .. (2 grain)
made or served with nonfat/low-fat milk	A B & C	1 cup .... (1 dairy)
Raisins	A	1 T .... (.5 fruit)
	B	2 T .... (1 fruit)
	C	4 T .... (2 fruit)
Walnuts in small pieces	A	2 T .... (1 nut)
	B & C	4 T .... (2 nut)
Coffee or tea with nonfat/low-fat milk	A B & C	½ cup .... (.5 dairy)

Note: Prepare tabouli salad for today's lunch and marinate chicken for dinner; refrigerate.

Meal #2

Morning Snack—Pear

Food	Plan	Serving
Pear	A B & C	1 pear .... (1 fruit)

Meal #3

Lunch—Tabouli Salad

Food	Plan	Serving
Tabouli Salad	A B & C	2 cups .... (2 grain, 2 vegetable, 2 oil)

For an easy-to-prepare version of this traditional Middle Eastern salad, look for a boxed version such as Fantastic Brand. Add 3 cups tomatoes and cucumbers (optional parsley, red bell pepper), 2 T olive oil, and lemon juice to taste. Serve on a bed of lettuce. Ready-to-serve versions of tabouli are available at many delis and natural food stores.

Meal #4

Afternoon Snack—Yogurt and Peaches

Food	Plan	Serving
Plain nonfat/low-fat yogurt	A	½ cup .... (.5 dairy)
	B & C	1½ cups .... (1.5 dairy)
Peach—sliced, fresh or frozen	A	¼ cup sliced ... (.5 fruit)
	B & C	½ cup sliced .. (1 fruit)

Meal #5

Dinner—COPIA Great Garden-Inspired Grilled Chicken with Couscous, Sun-dried Tomatoes, and Broccoli

(See recipe in Chapter 12.)

Food	Plan	Serving
COPIA great garden- inspired grilled chicken	A	3 oz .... (3 protein, 1 oil)
	B	5 oz .... (5 protein, 2 oil)
	C	5½ oz .... (5.5 protein, 3 oil)
Save extra for Day #8 dinner.		
Couscous (cooked)	A	½ cup .... (1 grain)
	B & C	1 cup .... (2 grain)
Sun-dried tomatoes (not in oil), chopped	A & B	1/3 cup .... (1 vegetable)
	C	2/3 cup .... (2 vegetable)
Broccoli—steamed, seasoned with lemon & salt	A B & C	1 cup .... (2 vegetable)
Today's pleasure foods	A	180 calories
	B	240 calories
	C	300 calories

Daily Meal Plan: Day #8

To substitute a food item, refer to the Daily Meal Plans Servings List on page 158.

Meal #1
Breakfast—Date Smoothie and Toast

Food	Plan	Serving	

Date smoothie —Mix in a blender

Food	Plan	Serving	
Nonfat or low-fat milk	A	¼ cup	(.25 dairy)
	B & C	½ cup	(.5 dairy)
Chopped and pitted dates	A & B	¼ cup	(1 fruit)
	C	½ cup	(2 fruit)
Banana	A	½ banana	(1 fruit)
	B & C	1 banana	(2 fruit)
Nonfat/low-fat plain yogurt	A	¼ cup	(.25 dairy)
	B & C	½ cup	(.5 dairy)
Optional	A B & C	½ cup ice	(free)
Toast	A B & C	1 slice	(1 grain)
with apple butter	A B & C	1 T	(free)
Coffee or tea with			
nonfat/or low-fat milk	A B & C	½ cup	(.5 dairy)

Meal #2
Morning Snack—Almonds

Food	Plan	Serving	
Almonds	A	2 T	(1 nut)
	B & C	4 T	(2 nut)

Meal #3
Lunch—Cheese Quesadilla

Food	Plan	Serving	
Cheese quesadilla:			
Whole-wheat tortilla(s)	A	1 tortilla	(1 grain)
	B & C	2 tortillas	(2 grain)

(80 calories or less per tortilla)

Mozzarella, part-skim	A	1½ oz	(1 dairy)
	B & C	2¼ oz	(1.5 dairy)

Spray skillet with cooking spray and cook until cheese melts or microwave 30 seconds.

Salsa	A B & C	¼ cup	(free)
Raw vegetables such as jicama and green, yellow, or red bell peppers	A B & C	1 cup	(2 vegetable)
V-8 or tomato juice (low sodium)	A B & C	6 oz	(1 vegetable)

Meal #4
Afternoon Snack—Popcorn

Food	Plan	Serving	
Popcorn, popped, no fat added or low-fat microwave	A B & C	3 cups	(1 grain)

Meal #5
Dinner—Mixed Green Salad with Chicken

Food	Plan	Serving	
Salad—mixed greens with tomatoes and cucumbers	A B & C	2 cups	(3 vegetable)
COPIA grilled chicken *(from Day #7 dinner)*			
	A	3 oz	(3 protein)
	B	5 oz	(5 protein)
	C	5½ oz	(5.5 protein)
Lemon & olive oil dressing	A	3 tsp	(3 oil)
	B	4 tsp	(4 oil)
	C	5 tsp	(5 oil)

(See recipe in Chapter 10.)

Sliced French or sourdough bread	A & B	1 slice	(1 grain)
	C	2 slices	(2 grains)

Spray with olive oil and toast under broiler.

Today's pleasure foods	A	180 calories	
	B	240 calories	
	C	300 calories	

Meal #1
Breakfast—Your Choice

Food	Plan	Serving
Protein serving(s)	A .... 1 serving	(1 protein)
	B & C .... 2 servings	(2 protein)
Grain serving(s)	A & B 1	(1 grain)
	C 2	(2 grain)
Dairy	A .... ¼ serving	(.25 dairy)
	B & C .... ¾ serving	(.75 dairy)
Coffee or tea with nonfat/low-fat milk	A B & C .... ¼ cup	(.25 dairy)

Meal #2
Morning Snack—Tangerine

Food	Plan	Serving
Tangerine	A & B .... 1 tangerine	(1 fruit)
	C .... 2 tangerines	(2 fruit)

Meal #3
Lunch—Vegetable and Tuna Pita Sandwiches
(See recipe in Chapter 10.)

Food	Plan	Serving
Vegetable and tuna filling	A .... 1 serving	(2 protein, .5 vegetable)
	B & C .... 1½ servings	(3 protein, .75 vegetable)
Whole-wheat pita bread	A B & C .... 1 pita	(2 grain)
Tomato, lettuce, sprouts	A .... 1 cup	(1 vegetable)
	B & C .... 2 cups	(2 vegetable)

Meal #4

Afternoon Snack—Baked Pear with Laughing Cow Cheese & Walnuts

(See recipe in Chapter 10.)

Food	Plan	Serving
Baked pear	A .... 1 pear .... (1 fruit)
	B & C .... 2 pears .... (2 fruit)
Laughing Cow Cheese— light	A B & C .... 2 wedges .... (1 dairy)
Chopped walnuts	A .... 2 T .... (1 nut)
	B & C .... 4 T .... (2 nut)

Meal #5

Dinner—Broccoli Soup and Bruschetta

(See recipes in Chapter 10.)

Food	Plan	Serving
Broccoli soup	A & B .... 1 serving .... (1.5 vegetable)
	C .... 2 servings .... (3 vegetable)

Make enough soup for tomorrow's lunch.

Food	Plan	Serving
Tomato and cheese bruschetta	A .... 1 bruschetta .... (1 grain, .5 vegetable, 1 oil, .5 dairy)
	B & C .... 2 brushettas .... (2 grain, 1 vegetable, 2 oil, 1 dairy)
Today's pleasure foods	A .... 180 calories
	B .... 240 calories
	C .... 300 calories

Daily Meal Plan: Day #10
To substitute a food item, refer to the Daily Meal Plans Servings List on page 158.

Meal #1

Breakfast—Waffles Topped with Strawberries and Yogurt

Food	Plan	Serving
Whole-wheat frozen waffles—toasted	A 1	(1 grain)
	B & C.................... 2	(2 grains)
Plain nonfat/low-fat yogurt	A .... ½ cup	(.5 dairy)
	B & C.................. 1 cup	(1 dairy)
Fresh or frozen sliced strawberries	A .... ½ cup	(1 fruit)
	B & C.................. 1 cup	(2 fruit)
Maple syrup (optional)	A B & C .... 1 T....................	50 pleasure food calories
Coffee or tea with nonfat/low-fat milk	A B & C .... ½ cup	(.5 dairy)

Meal #2

Morning Snack—Celery with Cottage Cheese

Food	Plan	Serving
Celery stalks	A .... 3 stalks............	(2 vegetable)
	B & C.................. 4 stalks............	(2+ vegetable)
Nonfat/low-fat cottage cheese	A .... ½ cup	(1 dairy)
	B & C.................. ¾ cup	(1.5 dairy)
Season with salsa	A B & C .... ¼ cup	(free)

Meal #3

Lunch—Broccoli Soup & Seasonal Vegetables

Food	Plan	Serving
Broccoli soup	A B & C .... 1 serving	(1.5 vegetable)

Use soup left over from yesterday.

Whole-wheat crackers
  (see box for serving size)   A & B .... 1 serving .... (1 grain)
                              C .... 2 servings .... (2 grain)

Seasonal vegetables   A & B .... 1 cup .... (1 vegetable)
                              C .... 1½ cups .... (1.5

                                                        vegetable)

Walnut oil dressing   A .... 3 tsp .... (3 oil)
                              B .... 4 tsp .... (4 oil)
                              C .... 5 tsp .... (5 oil)

(See recipe in Chapter 10.)

Walnuts–chopped   A .... 2 T .... (1 nut)
                              B & C .... 4 T .... (2 nut)

Meal #4
Afternoon Snack—Your Choice

Food	Plan	Serving
Fruit serving(s)	A & B .... 1 serving .... (1 fruit)	
	C .... 2 servings .... (2 fruit)	

Meal #5
Dinner—Lamb Chops, Sweet Potato, & Green Beans
(See recipe in Chapter 10.)

Food	Plan	Serving
Broiled lamb chops	A .... 3 oz .... (3 protein)	
	B .... 5 oz .... (5 protein)	
	C .... 5½ oz .... (5.5 protein)	
Baked sweet potato or yam	A B & C .... 2/3 cup .... (2 grain)	
Green beans—steamed,		
seasoned with lemon juice	A .... 1 cup .... (2 vegetable)	
	B & C .... 1½ cups .... (3 vegetable)	
Today's pleasure foods	A .... 180 calories	
	B .... 240 calories	
	C .... 300 calories	

Daily Meal Plan: Day #11
To substitute a food item, refer to the Daily Meal Plans Servings List on page 158.

Meal #1
Breakfast—Scrambled Eggs and Cheese with Bagel and Cream Cheese

Food	Plan	Serving
Whipped egg(s)	A	1 egg (1 protein)
	B & C	2 eggs (2 protein)
Nonfat/low-fat milk	A B & C	¼ cup (.25 dairy)
Mozzarella, part-skim cheese	A	¾ oz (.5 dairy)
	B & C	1½ oz (1 dairy)
Sliced red/green peppers	A	½ cup (1 vegetable)
	B & C	1 cup (2 vegetable)

Season with herbs, salt and pepper.

Food	Plan	Serving
Whole-wheat bagel	A	½ bagel (1 grain)
	B & C	1 bagel (2 grain)
with fat-free cream cheese	A B & C	1T (free)
100% fruit spread	A B & C	2 tsp (free if 20 or fewer calories)
Coffee or tea with nonfat/low-fat milk	A B & C	¼ cup (.25 dairy)

Meal #2
Morning Snack—Almonds

Food	Plan	Serving
Almonds	A	2 T (1 nut)
	B & C	4 T (2 nut)
Figs, raw	A	2 figs (1 fruit)
	B & C	4 figs (2 fruit)

Meal #3
Lunch—Your Choice

Food	Plan	Serving
Grain serving	A B & C	1 serving (1 grain)

Vegetable serving	A B & C .... 1+ serving .... (1+ vegetable)	
Dairy serving (s)	A .... 1 serving .... (1 dairy)	
	B & C .... 1½ servings .... (1.5 dairy)	

Meal #4
Afternoon Snack—Tangerine

Food	Plan	Serving
Tangerine	A & B .... 1 tangerine ..... (1 fruit)	
	C .... 2 tangerines .... (2 fruit)	

Meal #5
Dinner—California Cafe Angel Hair Pasta with Prawns
(See recipe in Chapter 12.)

Food	Plan	Serving
Angel Hair Pasta	A & B .... 1 cup .... (2 grains)	
	C .... 1½ cups .... (3 grains)	
Sauce	A & B .... ½ cup .... (1 vegetable)	
	C .... ¾ cup .... (1.5 vegetable)	
Prawns	A .... 2 oz .... (2 protein)	
	B .... 3 oz .... (3 protein)	
	C .... 3½ oz .... (3.5 protein)	
Mixed green salad	A .... 2 cups .... (2 vegetable)	
	B .... 2½ cups .... (2.5 vegetable)	
	C .... 3 cups .... (3 vegetable)	
Lemon and olive oil dressing	A .... 3 tsp .... (3 oil)	
	B .... 4 tsp .... (4 oil)	
	C .... 5 tsp .... (5 oil)	

(See dressing recipe in Chapter 10.)

Today's pleasure foods	A .... 180 calories	
	B .... 240 calories	
	C .... 300 calories	

If you choose to drink wine with dinner, suggested choices would be a Chardonnay or Sauvignon Blanc.

Daily Meal Plan: Day #12
To substitute a food item, refer to the Daily Meal Plans Servings List on page 158.

Meal #1
Breakfast—Oatmeal with Dates and Walnuts

Food	Plan	Serving
Oatmeal with cinnamon	A & B	½ cup cooked . (1 grain)
	C	¾ cup cooked . (1.5 grain)
with nonfat/low-fat milk	A B & C	½ cup .... (.5 dairy)
Dates—chopped and pitted	A & B	¼ cup .... (1 fruit)
	C	½ cup .... (2 fruit)
Walnuts—chopped	A	2 T .... (1 nut)
	C	4 T .... (2 nut)
Coffee or tea with nonfat/low-fat milk	A B & C	½ cup .... (.5 dairy)

Meal #2
Morning Snack—Your Choice

Food	Plan	Serving
Vegetable serving	A B & C	1 serving .... (1+vegetable)

Meal #3
Lunch—Greek Salad with Pita Bread
(See recipe in Chapter 10.)

Food	Plan	Serving
Greek Salad	A & B	1½ cups .... (1.5 vegetable)
	C	2 cups .... (2 vegetable)
Lemon and olive oil dressing	A	2 tsp .... (2 oil)
	B	2½ tsp .... (2 oil)
	C	3½ tsp .... (3.5 oil)
(See recipe in Chapter 10.)		
Feta cheese	A	½ oz .... (.5 dairy)
	B & C	1 oz .... (1 dairy)
Whole-wheat pita bread	A	½ .... (1 grain)
	B & C	1 .... (2 grain)

Meal #4
Afternoon Snack—Yogurt with Strawberries

Food	Plan	Serving
Nonfat/low-fat yogurt	A	½ cup .... (.5 dairy)
	B & C	1 cup .... (1 dairy)
Strawberries—sliced	A	½ cup .... (1 fruit)
	B & C	1 cup .... (2 fruit)

Meal #5
Dinner—Little River Inn Crab Cakes, Rice & Asparagus
(See recipe in Chapter 12.)

Food	Plan	Serving
Little River Inn crab cakes	A	1 patty .... (2.5 protein, .5 grain, .75 oil)
	B & C	2 patties .... (5 protein, 1 grain, 1.5 oil)

Save leftover cakes for lunch Day #14.

Food	Plan	Serving
Wild rice	A B & C	½ cup .... (1 grain)
Asparagus—steamed, seasoned with lemon, salt and pepper	A B & C	1 cup .... (2 vegetable)

Today's pleasure foods	A	180 calories
	B	240 calories
	C	300 calories

If you wish to have wine with your dinner, Riesling or Gewurztraminer would pair well with the crab cakes.

Begin marinating chicken for tomorrow night's Mediterranean Chicken. See Day #13.

Daily Meal Plan: Day #13

To substitute a food item, refer to the Daily Meal Plans Servings List on page 158.

Meal #1
Breakfast—Blueberry Smoothie and Toast

Food	Plan	Serving

Blueberry Smoothie—Mix in a blender.

Nonfat or low-fat milk	A	½ cup	(.5 dairy)
	B & C	1 cup	(1 dairy)
Fresh or frozen blueberries	A	1/3 cup	(.75 fruit)
	B & C	2/3 cup	(1.5 fruit)
Ice (optional)	A B & C	½ cup ice	(free)
Protein powder (optional)	A B & C	Use pleasure food calories	
Toast	A	1 slice	(1 grain)
	B & C	2 slices	(2 grains)
Apple butter on toast	A B & C	1 T	(free)
Coffee or tea with nonfat/low-fat milk	A B & C	¼ cup	(.25 dairy)

Meal #2
Morning Snack—Your Choice

Food	Plan	Serving
Dairy serving	A B & C	¾ serving	(.75 dairy)

Meal #3
Lunch—Hummus Salad Pita Sandwich

(See recipe in Chapter 10.)

Food	Plan	Serving
Whole-wheat pita bread	A B & C	1 whole pita	(2 grains)
Hummus	A & B	¼ cup	(.5 protein)
	C	½ cup	(1 protein)
Lettuce, tomato, sprouts, red peppers, lemon juice, salt, pepper to taste	A B & C	1 cup	(2 vegetable)

Feta cheese	A	½ oz	(.5 dairy)
	B & C	1 oz	(1 dairy)

Meal #4

Afternoon Snack—Baked Apple

(See recipe in Chapter 10.)

Food	Plan	Serving	
Baked apple	A & B	1	(1 fruit)
	C	2	(2 fruit)
Walnuts, chopped	A	1 T	(.5 nut)
	B & C	2 T	(1 nut)

Meal #5

Dinner—Fetzer Vineyards Mediterranean Chicken

(See recipe in Chapter 12.)
Save extra for Day #15 lunch.

Food	Plan	Serving	
Fetzer Vineyards Mediterranean Chicken			
Chicken	A	2½ oz	(2.5 protein)
	B & C	4½ oz	(4.5 protein)
Sauce	A	½ cup	(.25 fruit, 1.5 oil)
	B & C	1 cup	(.5 fruit, 3 oil)
Whole-grain couscous	A & B	½ cup	(1 grain)
	C	1 cup	(2 grain)
with toasted, sliced almonds	A	1 T	(.5 nut)
	B & C	2 T	(1 nut)
Steamed zucchini	A	1 cup	(2 vegetable)
	B & C	1½ cups	(3 vegetable)
Today's pleasure foods	A	180 calories	
	B	240 calories	
	C	300 calories	

If you wish to have wine with dinner, a Chardonnay or Viognier will pair well.

Meal #1

Breakfast—Spinach, Cheese, & Mushroom Omelet

(See recipe in Chapter 10.)

Food	Plan	Serving
Spinach, cheese, & mushroom omelet	A B & C	1 omelet .... (1 vegetable, 1 protein, .5 dairy)
Whole-wheat English muffin	A	½ muffin .... (1 grain)
	B & C	1 muffin .... (2 grain)
Coffee or tea with nonfat/low-fat milk	A B & C	¼ cup .... (.25 dairy)

Meal #2

Morning Snack—Orange

Food	Plan	Serving
Orange	A & B	1 orange.......... (1 fruit)
	C	2 oranges .... (2 fruit)

Meal #3

Lunch—Crab Cake Sandwich

Food	Plan	Serving
Crab cake *reheated from Day #12*	A	1 patty .... (2.5 protein, .5 grain, .75 oil)
	B & C	2 patties .... (5 protein, 1 grain, 1.5 oil)
French bread, sliced and toasted	A B & C	2 slices .... (2 grains)
spread with garlic/ ginger spread or nonfat mayonnaise	A B & C	1 T .... (free)
with lettuce, sprouts, tomato	A B & C	1 cup .... (1 vegetable)

V-8 or tomato juice   A B & C .... 6 oz .... (1 vegetable)
  This meal plan exchanges .5 dairy serving for .5 protein for A and C, and 1 dairy
serving for 1 protein for B.

Meal #4

Afternoon Snack—Peaches with Cottage Cheese

Food	Plan	Serving
Sliced peaches	A .... ½ cup .... (1 fruit)
	B & C .... 1 cup .... (2 fruits)
Nonfat/low-fat cottage cheese	A B & C .... ¼ cup .... (.5 dairy)

Meal #5

Dinner—Café La Haye Mache and Spring Vegetable Salad with Goat Cheese and Tapenade Toast

(See recipe in Chapter 12.)

Food	Plan	Serving
Spring vegetable salad	A & B .... 1 cup .... (2 vegetable)
	C .... 1½ cups .... (3 vegetable)
Goat cheese	A B & C .... ½ oz .... (.5 dairy)
Citrus vinaigrette	A & B .... 4 tsp .... (2 oil)
	C .... 6 tsp .... (3 oil)
Toast	A .... 1 slice .... (1 grain)
	B & C .... 2 slices .... (2 grain)
Tapenade	A .... 1¼ T .... (2.25 oil)
	B & C .... 2½ T .... (5 oil)

This meal plan exchanges 1 nut serving for 2 oil servings for A and 2 nut servings for 4 oil
servings for B and C.

Today's pleasure foods	A .... 180 calories
	B .... 240 calories
	C .... 300 calories

  If you wish to have wine with dinner, Chef John Reynolds suggests a Sauvignon Blanc
with this dish.

Daily Meal Plan: Day #15

To substitute a food item, refer to the Daily Meal Plans Servings List on page 158.

Meal #1
Breakfast—Your Choice

Food	Plan	Serving
Grain servings	A & B .... 1 serving .... (1 grain)	
	C .... 2 servings .... (2 grain)	
Protein servings	A .... 1 serving .... (1 protein)	
	B & C .... 2 servings .... (2 protein)	
Coffee or tea with nonfat/low-fat milk	A B & C .... ½ cup .... (.5 dairy)	

Meal #2
Morning Snack —Yogurt and Strawberries

Food	Plan	Serving
Yogurt	A .... ½ cup .... (.5 dairy)	
	B & C .... 1 cup .... (1 dairy)	
Strawberries	A .... 1/3 cup .... (.75 fruit)	
	B & C .... 2/3 cup .... (1.75 fruit)	

Meal #3
Lunch—Mediterranean Chicken Wrap

Food	Plan	Serving
Whole-wheat tortilla *(80 calories or less per tortilla)*	A B & C .... 1 tortilla .... (1 grain)	
Mediterranean chicken left over from dinner Day #13	A .... 2 oz................ (2 protein, 1 oil)	
	B & C .... 3 oz................ (3 protein, 1.5 oil)	
Sauce	A B & C .... ½ cup .... (.25 fruit, 1 oil)	
Green salad	A B & C .... 1 cup .... (2 vegetable)	
Café La Haye Vinaigrette *(See recipe in Chapter 12.)*	A & B .... 2 tsp .... (2 oil)	
	C .... 4 tsp .... (4 oil)	

Meal #4

Afternoon Snack—Baked Pear, Laughing Cow Cheese & Walnuts

(See recipe in Chapter 10.)

Food	Plan	Serving
Baked pear	A & B	1 pear .... (1 fruit)
	C	2 pears .... (2 fruit)
Laughing Cow Cheese light	A B & C	1 wedge .... (.5 dairy)
Chopped walnuts	A	2 T .... (1 nut)
	B & C	4 T .... (2 nut)

Meal #5

Dinner—Suit-Yourself Pizza

(See recipe in Chapter 10.)
Save a slice of this pizza for Day #16's lunch.

Food	Plan	Serving
Whole-wheat pizza crust	A	1/8 pizza .... (2 grains)
	B & C	1½ slices .... (3 grains)
Pizza sauce	A B & C	to cover crust .. (free)
Vegetables	A	½ cup .... (1 vegetable)
	B & C	1 cup .... (2 vegetable)
Mozzarella cheese, part skim	A	¾ oz .... (.5 dairy)
	B & C	1½ oz .... (1 dairy)
Crumbled feta cheese (optional)	A B & C	1 oz .... 75 pleasure food calories
Sliced kalamata olives (optional)	A B & C	1 olive .... 10 pleasure food calories
Today's pleasure foods	A	180 calories
	B	240 calories
	C	300 calories

Meal #1
Breakfast—Oatmeal with Walnuts

Food	Plan	Serving
Oatmeal, seasoned with cinnamon	A & B	½ cup cooked .. (1 grain)
	C...........................	1 cup cooked .. (2 grain)
with walnuts chopped	A	2 T.................... (1 nut)
	B & C..................	4 T.................... (2 nut)
with nonfat/low-fat milk	A B & C	½ cup .... (.5 dairy)
Coffee or tea with nonfat/low-fat milk	A B & C	½ cup .... (.5 dairy)

Meal #2
Morning Snack—Your choice

Food	Plan	Serving
Fruit serving(s)	A & B	1 serving .... (1 fruit)
	C...........................	2 serving .... (2 fruit)
Dairy serving	A	None
	B & C..................	½ serving .... (.5 dairy)

Meal #3
Lunch—Pizza and Salad

Food	Plan	Serving
Pizza—leftover from Day #15's dinner	A	1 slice .... (2 grain, 1 vegetable, .5 dairy)
	B & C	1½ slices .... (3 grain, 2 vegetable, 1dairy)

Plus any optional pleasure food calories from feta cheese or kalamata olives

Food	Plan	Serving
Mixed green with tomato salad	A	1 cup .... (1 vegetable)
	B	1½ cups .... (1.5 vegetable)
	C...........................	2 cups .... (2 vegetable)

Lemon and olive oil

    dressing   A .... 1 T .... (2.5 oil)

                            B .... 1½ T .... (4 oil)

                            C .... 2 T .... (5 oil)

(See recipe in Chapter 10.)

Meal #4
Afternoon Snack—Cantaloupe

<u>Food</u>	<u>Plan</u>	<u>Serving</u>
Cantaloupe—cubed	A .... ½ cup	(1 fruit)
	B & C .... 1 cup	(2 fruit)

Meal #5
Dinner—Italian Turkey Loaf
(See recipe in Chapter 10.)

<u>Food</u>	<u>Plan</u>	<u>Serving</u>
Italian turkey loaf	A .... 3½ oz	(3 protein, .5 vegetable)
	B .... 5½ oz	(5 protein, .75 vegetable)
	C .... 6 oz	(5.5 protein, 1 vegetable)
Save a slice for Day #17 lunch		
Steamed broccoli	A .... 1 cup	(2 vegetable)
	B .... 1½ cups	(3 vegetable)
	C .... 2 cups	(4 vegetable)
Baked potato, small	A B & C 1	(1 grain)
with nonfat/low-fat yogurt	A B & C .... ½ cup	(.5 dairy)
and salsa	A B & C .... ¼ cup	(free)
Today's pleasure foods	A .... 180 calories	
	B .... 240 calories	
	C .... 300 calories	

Daily Meal Plan: Day #17

To substitute a food item, refer to the Daily Meal Plans Servings List on page 158.

Meal #1
Breakfast—Fruit Smoothie

Food	Plan	Serving

Fruit smoothie—Mix in blender

Nonfat/low-fat milk	A	½ cup	(.5 dairy)
	B & C	1 cup	(1 dairy)
Orange juice	A	¼ cup	(.5 fruit)
	B & C	½ cup	(1 fruit)
Blueberries	A	¼ cup	(.5 fruit)
	B & C	½ cup	(1 fruit)
Protein powder (optional)	A B & C	Use pleasure food calories	
Whole grain English muffin	A & B	½ muffin	(1 grain)
	C	1 muffin	(2 grain)
with 100% fruit spread	A B & C	2 tsp	(free if 20 calories or less)
Coffee or tea with nonfat/low-fat milk	A B & C	½ cup	(.5 dairy)

Meal #2
Morning Snack—Almonds

Food	Plan	Serving

| **Almonds** | A | 2 T | (1 nut) |
| | B & C | 4 T | (2 nut) |

Meal #3
Lunch—Italian Turkey Loaf Sandwich

Food	Plan	Serving

Italian turkey loaf leftover from Day #16	A	3½ oz	(3 protein, .5 vegetable)
	B	5½ oz	(5 protein, .75 vegetable)
	C	6 oz	(5.5 protein, 1 vegetable)

Toasted Italian bread	A B & C	2 slices	(2 grains)
with ketchup	A B & C		(free)
Sliced bell peppers			
or green beans	A	1 cup	(2 vegetable)
	B & C	1½ cups	(3 vegetable)

Meal #4

Afternoon Snack—Your Choice

Food	Plan	Serving	
Fruit Serving(s)	A & B	1 serving	(1 fruit)
	C	2 servings	(2 fruit)
Dairy Serving	A B & C	½ serving	(.5 dairy)

Meal #5

Dinner—Penne Pasta

(See recipe in Chapter 10.)

Food	Plan	Serving	
Whole Grain Penne Pasta	A	1 serving	(1 grain, 1 vegetable, 1.5 oil)
	B & C	2 servings	(2 grains, 2 vegetable, 3 oil)
Kalamata olives	A	5 olives	(1 oil)
	B	8 olives	(1.5 oil)
	C	10 olives	(2 oil)
Crumbled feta cheese	A	½ oz	(.5 dairy)
	B & C	1 oz	(1 dairy)
Steamed spinach	A & B	½ cup	(1 vegetable)
	C	1 cup	(2 vegetable)
Today's pleasure foods	A	180 calories	
	B	240 calories	
	C	300 calories	

Daily Meal Plan: Day #18
To substitute a food item, refer to the Daily Meal Plans Servings List on page 158.

Meal #1
Breakfast—Fried Egg and Toast

Food	Plan	Serving	
Egg—fried with oil spray	A B & C	1 egg	(1 protein)
Toast	A	1 slice	(1 grain)
	B & C	2 slices	(2 grain)
Apple butter on toast	A B & C	1 T	(free)
Orange juice	A	½ cup	(1 fruit)
	B & C	1 cup	(2 fruit)
Coffee or tea with nonfat/low-fat milk	A B & C	½ cup	(.5 dairy)

Meal #2
Morning Snack—Cottage Cheese and Celery

Food	Plan	Serving	
Celery	A	½ cup	(1 vegetable)
	B & C	1 cup	(2 vegetable)
Non/low-fat cottage cheese	A	½ cup	(1 dairy)
	B & C	1 cup	(2 dairy)
with salsa	A B & C	¼ cup	(free)

Meal #3
Lunch—Turkey or Roast Beef

Food	Plan	Serving	
Sandwich or wrap			
Whole-wheat bread or tortilla	A B & C	2 slices	(2 grain)
(80 calories or less per tortilla)			
Sliced turkey or lean roast beef	A	2 oz	(2 protein)
	B	4 oz	(4 protein)
	C	4½ oz	(4.5 protein)
Sliced tomato, lettuce, sprouts, dill pickle	A	1 cup	(2 vegetable)
	B & C	2 cups	(4 vegetable)

Mozzarella cheese, part-skim	A B & C .... ¾ oz	(.5 dairy)
Mustard, horseradish sauce	A B & C	(free)

Meal #4

Afternoon Snack—Baked Apple with Walnuts

(See recipe in Chapter 10.)

Food	Plan	Serving
Baked apple	A &B 1	(1 fruit)
	C 2	(2 fruit)
Chopped walnuts	A .... 2 T	(1 nut)
	B & C .... 4 T	(2 nut)

Meal #5

Dinner—Wente Vineyards Tomato Soup

(See recipe in Chapter 12.)

Food	Plan	Serving
Wente Vineyards tomato soup	A .... 1 serving	(2.5 vegetable, 1 oil)
	B & C .... 2 servings	(5 vegetable, 2 oil)

Serve hot or cold depending on the season.

Whole grain sourdough bread, toasted	A & B .... 1 slice	(1 grain)
	C .... 2 slices	(2 grain)
Served with Café La Haye Tapenade leftover from Day #14 dinner	A & B .... 1 T...................	(2 oil)
	C .... 1½ T	(3 oil)
Garden greens salad	A B & C .... 2 cups	(2 vegetable)
Fat-free dressing	A B & C	(free)

(See dressing recipe in Chapter 10.)

Today's pleasure foods	A .... 180 calories
	B .... 240 calories
	C......................... 300 calories

If you wish to have wine with dinner, Chef Elisabeth Schwarz suggests serving Zinfandel.

Daily Meal Plan: Day #19

To substitute a food item, refer to the Daily Meal Plans Servings List on page 158.

Meal #1

Breakfast—Waffles, Yogurt, and Blueberries

Food	Plan	Serving	
Whole-wheat waffle	A	1 waffle	(1 grain)
	B & C	2 waffles	(2 grain)
Nonfat/low-fat yogurt	A	½ cup	(.5 dairy)
	B & C	1 cup	(1 dairy)
Blueberries, fresh or frozen	A & B	½ cup	(1 fruit)
	C	1 cup	(2 fruit)
Coffee or tea with nonfat/low-fat milk	A B & C	½ cup	(.5 dairy)

Meal #2

Morning Snack—Your Choice

Food	Plan	Serving	
Fruit serving(s)	A	1 serving	(1 fruit)
	B & C	2 servings	(2 fruit)
Nut serving(s)	A	2 T	(1 nut)
	B & C	4 T	(2 nut)
Dairy serving(s)	A	½ serving	(.5 dairy)
	B & C	1 serving	(1 dairy)

Meal #3

Lunch—Avocado Sandwich or Wrap

Food	Plan	Serving	
Whole-wheat bread or tortilla	A & B	1 slice	(1 grain)
	C	2 slices	(2 grain)
(80 calories or less per tortilla)			
Avocado	A & B	¼ avocado	(1.5 oil)
	C	1/3 avocado	(2 oil)
Mozzarella, part-skim	A B & C	¾ oz	(.5 dairy)
Lettuce, tomato, sprouts	A & B	1 cup	(1 vegetable)
	C	2 cups	(2 vegetable)

V-8 or tomato juice
low-sodium   A B & C .... 6 oz .... (1 vegetable)

Meal #4

Afternoon Snack—Crackers and Cream Cheese

Food   Plan   Serving

Whole-wheat crackers   A B & C .... 1 serving .... (1 grain)
   Note: Look on box for serving size.

Nonfat cream cheese   A B & C .... 1 T .... (free)

Jam or other topping
   (optional)   A B & C .... Use pleasure food calories

Meal #5

Dinner—Bouchon Santa Barbara Grilled Rosemary-Skewered Scallops

(See recipe in Chapter 12.)

Food   Plan   Serving

Rosemary skewered scallops A .... 6 scallops .... (3 protein,
                                                                1.5 oil)
                                B .... 10 scallops ...... (5 protein,
                                                                2.5 oil)
                                C .... 11 scallops .... (5.5 protein,
                                                                2.5 oil)

Grilled or steamed   A & B .... 1 cup .... (2 vegetable)
   asparagus   C .... 1½ cups .... (3 vegetable)

Risotto, whole grain   A B & C .... ½ cup .... (1 grain)

Today's pleasure foods   A .... 180 calories
                                B .... 240 calories
                                C .... 300 calories

If you wish to have wine with dinner, Bouchon Santa Barbara's proprietor, Mitchell Sjerven, suggests a Sauvignon Blanc or Pinot Noir. For more details see the recipe.

Daily Meal Plan: Day #20

To substitute a food item, refer to the Daily Meal Plans Servings List on page 158.

Meal #1
Breakfast—Kashi and Strawberries

Food	Plan	Serving
Kashi cereal	A & B	½ cup (1 grain)
	C	1 cup (2 grain)
Sliced strawberries	A	½ cup (1 fruit)
	B & C	1 cup (2 fruit)
Nonfat/low-fat milk	A	½ cup (.5 dairy)
	B & C	1 cup (1 dairy)
Coffee or tea with nonfat/low-fat milk	A B & C	½ cup (.5 dairy)

Meal #2:
Morning Snack—Almonds

Food	Plan	Serving
Almonds	A	2 T (1 nut)
	B & C	4 T (2 nut)

Meal #3
Lunch—Italian Sub Sandwich

Food	Plan	Serving
Turkey or pork sausage	A	3 oz (3 protein)
	B	5 oz (5 protein)
	C	5½ oz (5.5 protein)

Look for one of the new lean meat sausages that combines meat with vegetables.

Food	Plan	Serving
Red onion and green pepper, thinly sliced	A & B	1½ cups (3 vegetable)
	C	2 cups (4 vegetable)
Mozzarella, part-skim	A B & C	¾ oz (.5 dairy)

Spray sauté pan with olive oil and sauté onion and pepper until soft. Add sausage, top with cheese and heat until sausage is warm and cheese is melted.

Food	Plan	Serving
Serve on whole-wheat hot dog bun	A B & C	1 roll (2 grain)
with tomato sauce	A B & C	2 T (free)

V-8 or tomato juice,
  low-sodium   A B & C .... 6 oz .... (1 vegetable)

Meal #4
Afternoon Snack—Tangerine

Food   Plan   Serving

Tangerine   A & B .... 1 tangerine ..... (1 fruit)
                        C .... 2 tangerines .... (2 fruit)

Meal #5
Dinner—COPIA Polenta
and Grilled Vegetable Napoleons
(See recipe in Chapter 12)
Save leftovers for lunch Day #20.

Food   Plan   Serving

COPIA polenta   A .... 1 serving .... (1 grain,
                                                         1 vegetable, .5 oil, .5 dairy)
                        B & C .... 2 servings .... (2 grain,
                                                         2 vegetable, 1 oil, 1 dairy)
Basil vinaigrette   A .... 3 tsp .... (2.5 oil)
                        B .... 4 tsp .... (3 oil)
                        C .... 5 tsp .... (4 oil)

Today's pleasure foods   A .... 180 calories
                             B .... 240 calories
                             C .... 300 calories

If you wish to have wine with dinner, the creator of this dish, COPIA Culinary Instructor Jill Hough, suggests a White Zinfandel. For more details see the recipe.

Meal #1
Breakfast—Your Choice

Food	Plan	Serving
Grain serving	A B & C .... 1 serving	(1 grain)
Fruit serving	A & B .... 1 serving	(1 fruit)
	C.......................... 2 servings........	(2 fruit)
Protein	A B & C .... 1 serving	(1protein)
Coffee or tea with nonfat/low-fat milk	A B & C .... ½ cup	(.5 dairy)

Meal #2
Morning Snack—Cottage Cheese and Cantaloupe

Food	Plan	Serving
Nonfat/low-fat cottage cheese	A .... 1/3 cup.............	(.75 dairy)
	B & C.................. 2/3 cup.............	(1.5 dairy)
Cubed cantaloupe	A .... ½ cup	(1 fruit)
	B & C.................. 1 cup	(2 fruit)

Meal #3
Lunch—COPIA Polenta and Vegetable Napoleons
Reheated from Day #20 dinner

Food	Plan	Serving
Polenta	A & B .... 1½ servings	(1.5 grain, 1.5 vegetable, .75 oil, .75 dairy)
	C.......................... 2 servings........	(2 grain, 2 vegetable, 1 oil, 1 dairy)
Basil vinaigrette	A .... 2 tsp	(1.5 oil)
	B & C.................. 3 tsp	(2.5 oil)

Meal #4
Afternoon Snack—Sunflower Seeds

Food	Plan	Serving
Sunflower seeds	A	2 T (1 nut)
	B & C	4 T (2 nut)

Meal #5
Dinner—Los Olivos Café Oyster Salad

(See recipe in Chapter 12.)

Food	Plan	Serving
Oysters	A	4 oysters (.5 grain, 2 protein)
	B	8 oysters (1 grain, 4 protein)
	C	9 oysters (1 grain, 4.5 protein)
Vinaigrette	A & B	2 T (.75 oil)
	C	4½ T (1.5 oil)
Salad	A B & C	2 cups (3 veg)
Whole grain Italian bread	A	1 slice (1 grain)
	B	1½ slices (1.5 grain)
	C	2 slices (2 grain)
Today's pleasure foods	A	180 calories
	B	240 calories
	C	300 calories

If you wish to enjoy wine with dinner, Chef Nat Ely suggests Chenin Blanc or Chardonnay.

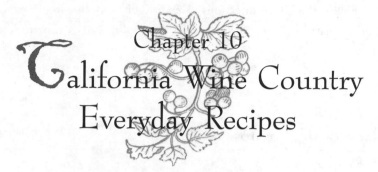

Chapter 10
California Wine Country Everyday Recipes

You don't have to cook fancy or complicated master-pieces—just good food from fresh ingredients.

—Julia Child

Breakfast

Spinach, Cheese, and Mushroom Omelet

Serves 1

1 egg

¾ oz mozzarella, part-skim cheese

¼ cup sliced mushrooms

1 cup fresh spinach, chopped or baby

(Optional: ½ cup nonfat/low-fat milk)

Whisk 1 egg (and milk if using it)

Coat an 8-inch skillet or omelet pan with cooking spray and heat over a medium heat. Sauté mushrooms, remove, and set aside. Spray pan again. Pour in the egg mixture. With a spatula lift the edges of the mixture to allow the uncooked portions to move underneath. Place the mushrooms, spinach, and cheese on top of the egg mixture. When it is set, fold the omelet over and serve.

Nutrition pyramid servings: 1 veg, 1 protein, .5 dairy (plus .5 dairy if using milk)

Suit-Yourself Vegetable Omelets

Follow the above directions using any of the following vegetables: onions, squash, bell peppers, artichoke hearts (in water), tomatoes, and asparagus.

Main Dishes

Black Bean Burritos

Serves 4

1½ tablespoons olive oil

1 carrot, sliced thinly

1 small onion, chopped

½ red bell pepper, sliced thinly

1 cup artichoke hearts in water, quartered

2 cups cleaned baby spinach

3 tablespoons cilantro

1 15-oz can black beans (rinsed well) or home-cooked

Salt to taste

½ teaspoon cumin

½ teaspoon chili powder

11/3 cups shredded mozzarella, part-skim

4 whole wheat tortillas (80 calories or less per tortilla)

1 tablespoon fat-free sour cream per serving

¼ cup salsa per serving

Sauté carrot, onion, and red bell pepper in oil for 2 minutes. Add spinach, artichoke hearts, cilantro, beans, and seasonings. Cook until spinach is wilted. Keep it warm as you heat tortillas on a non-stick skillet. Put vegetable mixture with 1/3 cup cheese in the middle of the warm tortilla. Fold over end and roll up. Serve with fat-free sour cream (1 tablespoon) and salsa.

Alternative: Use whatever vegetables are in the refrigerator.

Nutrition pyramid servings: 1 grain, 1.5 veg, 1.5 protein, 1 oil

Wine Country Broiled Lamb Chops

Serves 4

Preheat broiler.

Combine for 4 lamb chops:

1 tablespoon lemon juice

½ tablespoon minced garlic

½ tablespoon oregano

Salt and pepper to taste

Cover both sides of the lamb chops and place on a broiler pan that is covered with a cooking spray.

Broil approximately 4 minutes on each side. Thicker chops will take a little longer.

Nutrition pyramid servings: 1 protein per cooked ounce of lamb

Italian Turkey Loaf

This is a good meal to make ahead of time, to have ready to put in the oven when you get home. It's made with turkey but could also be made with lean beef.

Serves 8

1 tablespoon olive oil

½ onion chopped

½ red pepper chopped

2 stalks celery chopped

1 teaspoon dried thyme

1 teaspoon oregano

3 cloves garlic minced

½ teaspoon sea salt plus more for sautéing

¾ teaspoon fresh ground black pepper

1/8 teaspoon chili flakes

1 tablespoon tomato paste

6-8 ounces canned tomatoes chopped by hand or already diced

1 package lean ground turkey (1¼ pounds)

1 egg slightly beaten

¾ to 1 cup fresh bread crumbs

Spray a nonstick sauté pan with cooking spray. Use 1 tablespoon olive oil to sauté onions, pepper, and celery with sea salt for about 10 minutes, until soft. Add garlic and sauté a few more minutes until fragrant. To that add all the seasonings and sauté 1 minute more. Remove from heat and add the chopped tomatoes, their juice, and tomato paste. Taste for seasonings and add more salt/pepper/chile flakes as desired. The vegetable mixture should be cooled before adding it to the turkey mixture.

In another bowl, mix by hand the turkey with the egg and bread crumbs. Then add the cooled vegetable mixture. If you are making the recipe ahead of time, put this combined mixture into the refrigerator.

When you are ready for dinner, preheat the oven to 325 degrees. Place the turkey and vegetable mixture into a loaf pan that has been sprayed with cooking spray, or make a loaf shape and put the mixture directly onto a baking sheet.

Cook in the oven for 1 hour. It is done when an instant-read thermometer reads 160 degrees. Top with salsa.

Nutrition pyramid servings: .5 veg, 3 protein

Cajun Turkey Loaf

For a Cajun-style turkey loaf, follow the same directions as in the Italian version above but replace the spices with the following:

2 teaspoons paprika
2 teaspoons chili powder
1½ teaspoons dried oregano
½ teaspoon cumin
½ teaspoon salt
¼ teaspoon cayenne

Perfect Penne Pasta

Look for whole wheat or whole grain brown rice penne pasta. This is a vegetarian recipe but it is also very good with sliced Italian sausage.

Serves 8

8 dry ounces penne pasta (whole wheat or brown rice)
2 pounds fresh or canned tomatoes, halved, seeded, chopped
6 tablespoons chopped fresh parsley
¼ cup chopped fresh dill
1 cup chopped green onions (white and pale green parts only)
3 tablespoons olive oil
6 ounces crumbled feta cheese
20 black kalamata olives, pitted, and sliced

Cook pasta in a pot of boiling salted water until tender but still firm, approximately 5 to 7 minutes depending on the type of pasta.

Combine the remaining ingredients in a large bowl and set aside.

Drain the pasta and add to the tomato mixture. Toss to coat and put back in pan to warm up. Season to taste with salt and pepper.

Nutrition pyramid servings: 1 grain, 1 veg, 1.5 oil, .5 dairy

Suit-Yourself Pizza

This is a great meal for a busy night and one that will please everyone in the family. There are lots of good pizza dough recipes which you may want to try. Right now we're going to presume that you will be using a ready made pizza crust. Get a thin crust that is whole wheat if possible. Now the fun begins.

Serves 8

Cover the entire crust with pizza sauce.

You can cover the whole crust with the same toppings or have different people select their favorite toppings and put them on a specific area of the pizza.

For vegetables, grill or sauté them first in a pan using oil spray before putting them on the crust. Pile them as high as you like on your piece.

For those family members who are following the California Wine Country Diet, be sure to measure any cheese, olives, or meat that you put on their piece.

Here are ingredients for a "California Style" pizza: sun dried tomatoes, fresh diced garlic, fresh spinach, water packed artichoke hearts, fresh chopped cilantro, crumbled feta cheese, and pitted and chopped kalamata olives.

Follow the directions on the pizza crust package. Baking usually takes 5 to 10 minutes at 450 degrees, depending on how many toppings you have.

Nutrition pyramid servings: 1 slice (1/8 of the crust)= 2 grain, 1 veg per half cup added, 1 dairy per 1/3 cup grated mozzarella

Salads and Salad Dressings

Apple Walnut Salad

Serves 4

2 cups cored and cubed green apples

2 cups sliced celery

2 cups chopped red bell pepper

½ lemon

4 cups red leaf lettuce

Top with:

    Gorgonzola cheese (1ounce = 1 dairy serving)

    Shelled and chopped walnuts (2–4 tablespoons)

Cover apples with lemon juice immediately after cutting to prevent browning. Mix and toss with celery and red bell pepper. Pour dressing (see below) over apple mixture and toss until coated.

Make a bed of 1 cup of lettuce on dinner plates. Place 1½ cups of mixture on lettuce bed. If you are on Plan A, sprinkle 2 tablespoons of walnuts and 1 ounce of cheese on top. If you are on Plan B, sprinkle 4 tablespoons of walnuts and 1½ ounces of cheese on top.

Nutrition pyramid servings: 1 fruit, 2 veg, Plan A: 1 nut and 1 dairy; Plan B: 2 nut and 1.5 dairy

Apple Walnut Salad Dressing

½ cup plain low-fat yogurt

¼ cup apple cider vinegar

1 tablespoon grainy mustard

1 tablespoon chopped shallots

1 garlic clove

1 tablespoon fresh basil leaves

Put ingredients in a blender and blend until smooth.
Nutrition pyramid servings: Free

Fat-Free Dressing

½ cup balsamic vinegar

3 tablespoons orange juice

3 tablespoons water

3 tablespoons nonfat mayonnaise

¼ teaspoon dried basil

¼ teaspoon dried oregano

¼ teaspoon salt

¼ teaspoon sugar or sugar substitute

Whisk the ingredients together until well blended.
Nutrition pyramid servings: Free

Greek Salad

Serves 4

2 medium tomatoes, sliced

4 cups romaine lettuce, torn into bite-sized pieces

½ cup cucumber, sliced thinly

½ cup red onion, sliced thinly

1 cup bell peppers—red, green, or yellow—sliced thinly

1 tablespoon minced fresh Italian (flat-leaf) parsley

½ cup feta cheese, sprinkled on top

Optional: 5 pitted and sliced kalamata olives for 1 oil serving or 45 pleasure food calories.

Nutrition pyramid servings: 1.5 veg, .5 dairy

Lemon and Olive Oil Dressing

¼ cup extra virgin olive oil
1 tablespoon fresh lemon juice
1 clove minced garlic
½ teaspoon minced fresh oregano or
¼ teaspoon crushed dried oregano

Whisk ingredients together, measure for each serving, and toss individual salads just before serving.

Nutrition pyramid servings: 1 tablespoon = 2.5 oil

Healthful Hummus

Serves 6

1 can garbanzo beans (drain and save the juice)
2 tablespoons sesame tahini
3 teaspoons lemon juice
3 peeled small (or 1 large) garlic cloves
½ teaspoon salt
¼ teaspoon pepper

Add all ingredients to a food processor and process until smooth.

Mix in the saved juice to get desired consistency. Experiment with different spices.

Nutrition pyramid servings: 1.5 protein, .5 nuts

Seasonal Vegetables with Walnuts

Serves 1

Cut up your favorite fresh, seasonal vegetables (or whatever is in the refrigerator or pantry) and fill at least 1 cup. This could include tomatoes, carrots, celery, shelled peas, pea pods, radishes, cooked vegetables from previous meals, and artichoke hearts (in water). Use your imagination.

Place the vegetables in a bowl with amount of walnuts according to your calorie plan and toss. Serve individually with Walnut Oil Dressing according to your calorie plan. If you are unable to find walnut oil, olive oil may be substituted.

Nutrition pyramid servings: 1 veg, 1–2 nut

Walnut Oil Dressing

1/3 cup walnut oil

½ teaspoon mustard

½ teaspoon dried tarragon

Salt and pepper to taste

Blend ingredients together.

Nutrition pyramid servings: 1 tablespoon = 3 oil

Sandwiches

Vegetable and Tuna Salad Pita Sandwiches

Serves 3

Combine the following in a bowl and mix well:

1 6½ ounce can of tuna in spring water, drained

3 tablespoons fat-free mayonnaise

3 green onions, finely chopped

3 tablespoons celery, finely chopped

2 tablespoons parsley, finely chopped

3 tablespoons green pepper, finely chopped

2 tablespoons salsa

Pepper, freshly ground to taste

Put ingredients into half of a wholewheat pita with a tomato slice, lettuce, and alfalfa sprouts.

Nutrition pyramid servings: .5 veg, 2 protein

Tomato and Cheese Bruschetta

Crostini evolved in Italy, it is said, as a way to deal with stale bread. Basically you can put on any topping you wish from tomatoes and basil to smoked salmon with mozzarella melted on top. Always start with a good quality, dense, country-style bread such as a baguette. Bruschetta is the simplest form of Crostini, in which the bread is toasted on both sides and then topped with fresh garlic and olive oil.

Serves 1
2 slices Italian bread
1 medium tomato, seeded and chopped
2 teaspoons sliced basil
2 teaspoons olive oil
1 small garlic clove, minced
Salt and pepper to taste
1.5 oz Mozzarella, part-skim cheese

Combine tomato, basil, garlic, olive oil, salt, and pepper. Toast bread lightly. Spray both sides with olive oil. Spread half of the mixture on the toast. Top with cheese. Bake in upper half of oven at 400 degrees for 5 to 7 minutes or until cheese melts.

Nutrition pyramid servings: 2 grain, 1 veg, 2 oil, 1 dairy

MISTO Bruschetta*

"Slice a loaf of fresh Italian bread about ¾" thick. Toast lightly, and spray both sides with garlic-flavored olive oil. Spread a tablespoon of salsa on the toast then layer a few slices of fresh roasted peppers and plum tomatoes. Dust them with parmesan cheese and broil until cheese browns."

Serving size: 1 slice of bread with 1/8 cup parmesan cheese
Nutrition pyramid servings: 1 grain, .5 veg, .5 dairy

Recipe reprinted with the permission of Liquid Motion, Inc. More recipes using the MISTO sprayer can be found at www.misto.com.

Soups

Broccoli Soup

Serves 4
6 cups broccoli
1 carton (1 quart) chicken or vegetable broth
½ teaspoon salt
¼ teaspoon ground pepper
2 tablespoons lemon juice
Optional: ¾ oz mozzarella part-skim cheese per serving

Heat broth in a large saucepan to simmering and add chopped broccoli. Simmer in the covered pot for 15 minutes until broccoli is tender.

You can puree the soup with a blender or food processor. The easiest way is with an immersion blender, which you can use right in the saucepan.

Season with salt, pepper, and lemon juice. Sprinkle with cheese if you wish.

Nutrition pyramid servings: 1.5 veg, .5 dairy if cheese is used

Cauliflower and Roasted Red Pepper Soup

Follow the same directions as for the broccoli soup but use 5 cups cauliflower and add 1 cup sliced, roasted red bell peppers after 10 minutes of cooking. You can buy roasted red bell peppers in jars in the gourmet section of many supermarkets. Makes a great soup with a light spicy taste.

Snacks

Baked Apple

Serves 1
1 apple per person
Cinnamon
Optional: 2-4 tablespoons chopped walnuts
Optional: 1 teaspoon butter

Peel and core your favorite type of apple. Cut into 6 slices.

Place in a microwave-safe dish. Sprinkle with cinnamon.

Cover dish with paper towel. Cook for 3 minutes and then check to see if it is done.

Nutrition pyramid servings: 1 fruit, 1-2 nut if walnuts are used, 33 pleasure food calories if butter is used

Baked Pear

Serves 1

1 pear

Cinnamon

1 wedge Laughing Cow light cheese

Peel and core your favorite type of pear. Cut into 4 slices.

Place in a microwave-safe dish. Place Laughing Cow cheese on top of pear. Sprinkle with cinnamon. Cover with paper towel. Cook in microwave for 2 minutes and then check to see if it is done.

Nutrition pyramid servings: 1 fruit, .5 dairy

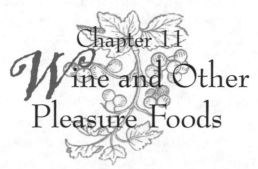

Chapter 11
Wine and Other Pleasure Foods

"My view, and that of many doctors with whom I've shared it, is that otherwise healthy people without contraindications for wine are highly likely to enhance their pleasure by enjoying wine in moderation with everyday dinner, and may strengthen their physical health in the process." —Andrea Immer, Master Sommelier

Now that you have your daily food plans for three weeks and know what to eat to fulfill your basic daily nutritional requirements, we have arrived at the top of the nutrition pyramid. This tier is called "Pleasure Foods," which are measured by calories rather than by servings, to give you the most flexibility in selection. You can use up to 15 percent of your daily calories for pleasure foods. For the 1,200-calorie Plan A that would be 180 calories. For the 1,600-calorie Plan B, you are allowed 240 calories. For the 2,000-calorie Plan C, the allowance is 300 calories a day. While you will eventually be choosing all the foods you eat, the pleasure food calories are there to give you freedom from the beginning to choose those extras that are not necessary nutritionally or are above your daily food-group serving limits.

When limiting your calories on a diet, it is especially important to pay careful attention to meeting your nutritional needs. As has been pointed out before, pleasure foods satisfy your emotional, basic self. Completely denying yourself the foods you love is a surefire way to derail all your good intentions for losing weight, because you will expend too much emotional energy trying to be "good." Sooner or later your basic self will rebel.

Likewise, following an extremely strict dietary regime almost en-sures that you will not be making long-term changes, but simply biding your time until you lose the weight and can go off the diet.

If an outside authority tells you *exactly* what to eat throughout a diet, you will not know what to do yourself once you are off it.

As you have discovered, the California Wine Country Diet pro-gram is different. You will have the choice of pleasure foods from the first day of the program and so can satisfy, albeit in a tempered way, the needs of your basic self. In addition, with each succeeding week you will be given an increasing number of choices for your other food selections, until by the fourth week you are designing your own meals using the serving guidelines you have learned. This program is about self-empower-ment, with you making the commitment *and* the decisions, based on your unique lifestyle needs.

Conscious Indulgence

Conscious indulgence is your mantra. Always be aware of how much you allow yourself to indulge your basic desires. You can calculate your daily pleasure food calories any number of ways: by using the calorie list that comes later in this chapter, consulting a calorie-counting book, or reading food labels.

My hope is that as time goes by you will increasingly choose plea-sure foods that are also healthy for you. This, however, is your choice. Perhaps your greatest love is jelly donuts, and having one every day will help keep you on track. I would still urge you to consider trying some dark chocolate instead, which is not only rich in taste but rich in antioxi-dants. But you always have the final say in which pleasure foods you choose to include in your meal plans.

Conscious Indulgence and Special Occasions

While your goal is to stay within your daily calorie limit, in the real world there are times when you will eat or drink more than that limit—a special meal out, holidays, potlucks, a wine-tasting tour, vacations. The biggest difference between thin people and heavy people often is what they do *after* they overeat. The thin person is likely to say, "I had a big

Thanksgiving dinner yesterday, so I'm going to eat lightly today." The overweight, and often dieting, person is more likely to instantly place blame on himself or herself and use that as an excuse to give up: "Now I've really done it! I've blown this diet. I'm so weak. I might as well just eat what I want to until I'm ready to be disciplined about losing weight."

Part of conscious indulgence, therefore, is to counter occasional overeating with a *little* under-eating. I am not talking about starving or severely restricting yourself all day and then binge eating at night. That is a common compulsive overeating pattern. What I am talking about is perhaps postponing some of your protein and grain servings during the day if you are going out that night for a restaurant meal. Or on Thanksgiving Day, you might wake up late and have brunch instead of breakfast and lunch before you head off to the family's traditional feast. While most of the time you will eat in a consistent pattern spaced throughout the day, you need the flexibility to be able to enjoy special occasions without the guilt that leads to discouragement and feelings of defeat.

Conscious Indulgence, Overeating, Compulsive Overeating, and Addiction

It is primarily in the area of pleasure foods that we have concerns about overeating, compulsion, and addiction. The ideal way to eat is to consume all food groups in moderation. However, I have learned in my years of working with people who have eating disorders and weight problems that many people have compulsive and addictive patterns with certain types of foods and alcohol. The question of whether this stems from food allergies, emotional problems, hormonal imbalances, or other causes is beyond the province of this book. We will focus, instead, on how to best deal with these patterns.

To see where you may fall on the conscious indulgence/overeating/compulsive overeating/addiction scale, we are going to shift over to the California Wine Country Diet practicality pyramid to analyze the underlying dynamics of the pattern.

For our pleasure food, let us choose potato chips, which are a challenge for most of us to eat in moderation. Imagine that you are just home from work, tired and hungry. You look around the kitchen for something quick to eat. On the counter is an apple and a bag of potato chips. You have a decision to make.

The first tier of the practicality pyramid is "Cooperation," although this is a place where your basic and conscious selves are often in competition instead of cooperation. Your conscious self remembers from reading those calorie-counting books that an apple weighs approximately 3.5 ounces and has 43 calories, with only a trace of fat and 11 grams of carbohydrate. Your conscious self thinks that sounds like an excellent choice. Then your basic self says, "Oh, but those potato chips look so good and we haven't used any pleasure food calories today." Your conscious self looks on the package and reads that in 1.4 ounces of the chips, there are 204 calories, 13 grams of fat, including 5.3 grams of saturated fats, and 21 grams of carbohydrate. The negotiation between the basic and conscious self is in full swing.

The second tier of the practicality pyramid is "Observation." So, a part of you moves into witnessing mode as you now observe what you do with this apple verses potato chip choice. There are many possibilities for this scenario to play itself out, but we will consider the three most common ones.

In Scenario 1, your conscious self suggests that you bake the apple in the microwave with cinnamon and a dab of butter so that you do not use up any of your pleasure food calories but still have a delicious snack quickly. Your basic self likes the idea, and so you enjoy a healthy snack and save your pleasure food calories for a glass of wine and piece of chocolate later on. You are *consciously indulging* through cooperation between your conscious and basic selves.

In Scenario 2, your basic self holds out for the potato chips. You carefully measure 1.4 ounces of potato chips on a small plate and eat them one by one with great delight. You accept your conscious self's acknowledgment that you have just used up all of your pleasure food calories for the day, and so for tonight you will have to forgo the glass of wine you so enjoy with dinner. You are aware of consciously indulging your basic self.

In Scenario 3, you do not think much about your choice, tear open the bag of chips and munch away, denying the fact that you are mindlessly eating more than 408 calories. You are overeating, not consciously indulging. Your basic self has taken control and you are not practicing either Cooperation or Observation.

If you take Scenario 3 one step further, you sneak the potato chips into the bedroom, where no one will catch you. Then you consume the whole bag, even though you are feeling full after only half the bag. You are in a compulsive overeating pattern. If you eat potato chips this way often and find it impossible to eat them in moderation, you are in an addictive pattern.

It pays off in the long run to spend some time at the beginning of any diet program or nutritional lifestyle change looking at where you are in relationship to your favorite pleasure foods and beverages. Doing so will provide vital information that will contribute to your success on the California Wine Country Diet program.

Conscious Indulgence to Addiction Scale

List your favorite pleasure foods/beverages under the categories of the following conscious indulgence to addiction continuum according to how easy or difficult it is for you to limit the amount you consume.

Food or Beverage

I consciously indulge: _____

I overeat: _____

I compulsively overeat: _____

I am addicted to: _____

Having taken an honest assessment of your relationship to different pleasure foods, it is time to move to the next tier of the practicality pyramid, which is "Acceptance." Accepting what your patterns are is not easy, especially when it might mean giving up your favorite treats. Without this acceptance, however, any weight loss and maintenance program will fail. Once you have accepted your patterns with compassion and without judgment, you will be free to move onto tier 4 "Choosing."

If you listed a treat under the conscious indulgence heading in the continuum above, you should have no problem including this food in your meal plans. If you listed a treat as being one that you tend to overeat, you have the choice of always weighing and measuring that food or not including it in your meal plans, at least not at the start of the program. However, if you faithfully measure your portions and consciously avoid allowing your portions to creep up, you will easily be able to move that food from the overeating to the conscious indulgence category.

The foods you listed under the compulsive overeating heading pose a greater challenge. These are the foods that, if they are in the house or on the table at work, you just cannot stop eating. The easiest strategy to deal with this compulsion is to not allow these foods to be in your environment at all. If you really want to continue eating them, then you will have to be extremely conscious about allowing yourself only an individual portion, and keep the larger portions out of sight. You will need to be honest with yourself, and you will need to call up your self-discipline and willpower. Can you really do this? There are more factors to answering this question than you may think. For instance, for people affected by seasonal depression, this strategy may work well in the spring and summer but not in the fall and winter. Women dealing with monthly hormonal changes may find that they compulsively overeat when premenstrual. The key to answering this question honestly is to consciously observe yourself and genuinely accept your feelings and behaviors. Only then can you make truly conscious choices.

Finally, we come to the foods or beverages you are addicted to. Depending on how this addiction is impacting your life, often complete abstinence is your only wise choice. Other times, you can cut down or substitute healthier alternatives. My experience in this field reveals that knowledge is power. When I work with individual clients, we first spend time discovering what is most appealing about the food or beverage they are addicted to. Then we try to find alternative ways to meet these "pleasure" needs while slowly or completely giving up the addiction.

As an example, "George" was addicted to a popular soda, and he drank at least two two-liter bottles a day. He was consuming more than 1,500 calories just from soda. He disliked diet soda, so you can imagine that weight loss would be nearly impossible with this pattern. As we discussed what was so appealing about soda, George discovered it was not the taste as much as it was the coldness of the beverage and the carbonation that satisfied him. Once we knew that, we were quickly able to come up with a number of far healthier and less fattening alternative beverages that he could drink, like sparkling water, which comes in flavors such as raspberry, lemon, and lime. George tried the alternatives, learned to enjoy several, and stopped drinking soda. He then was finally able to lose and to maintain a healthy weight.

Enjoying the Pleasure of All Foods

Before we start looking at where you might want to spend your pleasure food calories it is important to reflect on what we have been saying throughout the book—that all your food can and should be pleasurable. Not only are you looking for foods that are nutrient dense, but ones which are fresh and tasty also. When you wake up in the morning wouldn't you rather have one piece of exceptionally tasty raisin-walnut whole-wheat bread made by a local bakery than suffer through two pieces of reduced calorie bread that taste like cardboard? It takes just a few seconds more to look for that special piece of fruit or vegetable. Then as we talked about in Chapter 4 Pleasure, take the time to really enjoy eating. The more you enjoy all the food you eat, the less important the pleasure food calories will be. All of your calories will be pleasure calories.

Enjoying the Pleasure of Extra Servings

Especially when you are starting out on the California Wine Country Diet you may want to use many of your pleasure food calories for extra servings of the basic food groups. If you are coming from a high-protein diet, you may want to use your extra calories for more fish or meat. You may want to have two salads in a day and use more calories for olive oil. Perhaps you want to make a whole-wheat crust for a pizza and need more grain servings. The extra calories are also useful when you are eating out and cannot measure exactly what is in your dish. Enjoy the process of selecting how you are going to spend your extra calories. Remember that you are establishing a lifetime eating pattern that will lead to better health and a more enjoyable life.

Enjoying the Pleasure of Saturated Fat

As we talked about in Chapter 1 Nutrition, saturated fats, along with hydrogenated fats and trans-fatty acids, should be consumed sparingly because ingesting too much has been shown to raise LDL-cholesterol. We also want to monitor our fat intake because, calorie for calorie, fat has more than twice as many calories as protein or carbohydrate for its weight.

To give up all saturated fats would mean giving up such appealing foods as bacon, butter, coconut, cream, half and half, cream cheese, shortening, and sour cream. Then there are our old favorites, which include both saturated fats and refined sugar: pies, cakes, cookies, quiche, ice cream, and most candies. As we have talked about so many times in the *California Wine Country Diet,* the trick to enjoying these foods in a healthful way is to limit our intake of them to consciously indulge in them.

You, and only you, are making the choices of how you want to spend your pleasure food calories. If having two tablespoons of half and half with two teaspoons of sugar in your morning coffee is one of your greatest enjoyments in life, then perhaps you will want to spend 70 calories on your coffee. Or you might decide to switch to a latté with a half cup of low-fat milk and a sugar substitute. That will cost you only one-half of your allotted low-fat milk serving, and you can save those 70 calories for later, perhaps for a chocolate-chip cookie snack. The choice is yours, but make your choice a conscious one.

Chocolate, A Health Food?

For many of us, chocolate is a temptation that is nearly impossible to resist. Despite its popularity, chocolate is often one of the first foods to be eliminated by people trying to lose weight because of its high calorie content. Although it has long been considered a fattening and "empty" food, there is mounting evidence that chocolate actually has a number of health benefits. Researchers are finding many reasons to consider that chocolate in moderation can be part of a well-rounded diet.

Chocolate contains essential trace elements and nutrients such as iron, copper, calcium, and potassium, and such vitamins as A, B_1, C, D, and E. Cocoa is also the highest natural source for magnesium, which is beneficial for the cardiovascular system and hypertension. Adding magnesium (i.e., via chocolate) to one's diet has been proven to increase premenstrual progesterone levels. It is the drop in these levels that is responsible for the mood swings that are familiar to so many women. While chocolate is high in fat, it is not the type of fat that increases cholesterol levels. And dark chocolate contains high levels of flavonoid antioxidants, which have been proven to help inhibit heart disease, stimulate the immune system, and impede cancer growth. In fact, dark chocolate is believed to contain eight times the level of antioxidants found in strawberries. It also is believed to release endorphins in the brain, which help to elevate mood and reduce pain.[1, 2]

However, all these benefits do not free us to overindulge in chocolate. Here are some considerations for sensibly enjoying the pleasure of chocolate:

- Your healthiest choices of chocolate are high-quality dark chocolate or bittersweet chocolate containing a minimum of 70 percent or more cocoa solids. The intense flavors may also help you eat less.
- Stay away from "commercial" chocolates, which are low (less than 20 percent) in chocolate solids and high in sugar and saturated fats. A small candy bar weighs in at about 200 calories, with 50 percent coming from fat.
- Eat chocolate for dessert rather than as a snack. You are more likely to eat less of it if you consume it after finishing a satisfying meal.
- You can easily satisfy a chocolate craving and save calories by dipping fruit into melted dark chocolate or having a cup of reduced-sugar hot cocoa.
- Cut your favorite chocolate into ½ ounce (70 calorie) serving sizes and wrap them individually. Then enjoy the rapture of chocolate by letting one piece slowly melt in your mouth. Increase your pleasure even more by drinking red wine with your chocolate.

Favorite Pleasure Foods

The following list will give you an approximate idea of the calorie content of many favorite pleasure foods. Since there is such variation by brand and type in processed foods, for the most accurate calculation of calories in your favorite pleasure foods consult package labels and/or a book that lists calories.[3] Make sure to note the serving size used.

Food/Beverage	Serving Size	Calories
Avocado	½ cup	121
Bacon	2 slices	80
Bagel	2 ounces	157
Beer—regular	12 fluid ounces	146
Beer—light	12 fluid ounces	100
Biscuit—buttermilk	2 ounces	200
Bread	1 slice	100
Brownie	1 piece	150
Butter	1 tablespoon	100
Butterscotch topping	2 tablespoons	130
Cake	1/8 cake	300
Hershey's Kisses	1.3 ounces	160
Chocolate—dark or bittersweet	1.4 ounces	220
Chocolate syrup	2 tablespoons	110
Cocoa	1 tablespoon	30
Cocoa mix—fat-free	3 tablespoons	50
Cheese blue/cheddar/Monterey Jack	1 ounce	110
Cheese feta/goat/Mozzarella	1 ounce	80
Cheese Ricotta—whole milk	¼ cup	100
Cheese Ricotta—nonfat milk	¼ cup	50
Cheesecake	1 piece	190
Coconut	1 ounce	100
Coconut—flaked	2 tablespoons	70
Coffee iced—café latte	8 fluid ounces	130
Coffee—cappuccino	9.5 fluid ounces	190
Cookie—oatmeal	1.1 ounce	120
Cookie—chocolate chip	.9 ounce	140
Cookie—peanut butter	1.4 ounce	200

Cookie—fudge	1 ounce	150
Corn chips	1.1 ounces	140
Crackers	.5 ounces	60
Cream	1 tablespoon	45
Cream, half and half	2 tablespoons	40
Cream, whipping, heavy	1 tablespoon	50
Cool Whip	2 tablespoons	25
Cool Whip—fat free	2 tablespoons	15
Croissant	2.75 ounces	290
Danish	4.5 ounces	470
Donut	2 ounces	210
Granola	½ cup	225
Granola bar	1 bar	140
Guacamole	2 tablespoons	60
Honey	1 tablespoon	60
Hummus	2 tablespoons	60
Ice cream—Ben & Jerry's Wavy Gravy	½ cup	340
Ice cream—Healthy Choice Brownie	½ cup	110
Jelly	1 tablespoon	50
Liquor—80 proof	1 fluid ounce	64
Liquor—90 proof	1 fluid ounce	73
Liquor—100 proof	1 fluid ounce	82
Mayonnaise	1 tablespoon	100
Mayonnaise—light	1 tablespoon	50
Mayonnaise—fat-free	1 tablespoon	10
Milk—whole	1 cup	150
Milk—1%	1 cup	100
Muffin, blueberry	1.5 ounces	130
Muffin, English	1 whole	120
Oil	1 tablespoon	120
Olives—black	10 extra large	89
Orange juice	8 ounces	110
Pizza—deep dish	¼ of 12-" pie, cheese	375

Pizza—thin crust	¼ of 12" pie, cheese	273
Peanuts dry/honey roasted	1 ounce	160
Peanut butter	2 tablespoons	200
Pesto sauce, refrigerated	¼ cup	290
Pesto sauce—light	¼ cup	230
Pie—apple	1/8 pie	370
Popcorn—Newman's Own Butter Boom	3½ cups	170
Popcorn—Newman's Own Light	3½ cups	110
Potato baked in skin	1 medium	220
Potato—hash browns	1 cup	70
Potato chips	1 ounce	150
Potato, sweet	5" x 2" potato	118
Pretzels	1 ounce	110
Pudding	4 ounces	140
Pudding—fat-free	4 ounces	100
Pumpkin seeds	1 ounce	127
Ravioli	4.5 ounces	210
Salad dressing—Newman's Own Italian	2 tablespoons	120
Salad dressing—Newman's Own Italian Light	2 tablespoons	45
Salad Dressing—Wishbone Italian Fat-Free	2 tablespoons	10
Sausage—beef	2 links	170
Sausage—chicken	2 links	160
Sausage—pork	3 links	190
Sherbet	½ cup	130
Sherbet bar	1 bar	50
Sherbet bar—no sugar	1 bar	25
Snack mix—Chex Bold Party Blend	1 ounce	140
Soft drinks—club soda	12 ounces	0
Soft drinks—Coca Cola/Pepsi	12 ounces	100
Soft drinks—Orange Slice	12 ounces	190
Soy beverage	8 ounces	110
Soy beverage—light	8 ounces	60

Sugar	1 teaspoon	15
Sunflower seeds	1 ounce	180
Tabouli	½ cup	160
Tofu fresh/firm	½ cup	70
Tomato—sun-dried	1 ounce	73
Wine—dessert	5 ounces	226
Wine —red	5 ounces	106
Wine—white	5 ounces	100
Yogurt—plain/low fat	8 ounces	130
Yogurt—plain/non fat	8 ounces	100
Yogurt, frozen, Ben & Jerry's Phish Food	½ cup	230
Yogurt—frozen, Ben & Jerry's Cherry Garcia	½ cup	170
Yogurt—frozen, Dreyer's Chocolate Fudge Fat-Free	½ cup	100

Before you go any further in this chapter, take the time to make a list of the calories in your favorite pleasure foods. Read the labels for serving sizes and calorie counts. Review the list you made earlier in this chapter for your favorite pleasure foods on the Conscious Indulgence to Addiction scale. Now is a good time to decide which pleasure foods to continue enjoying and which ones it is wisest to avoid. Make a list in the form below and refer to it when you are choosing your daily pleasure foods.

My Pleasure Foods

Food/Beverage   **Serving Size**   **Calories**

_____

_____

_____

_____

_____

_____

The Pleasure of Wine

The drinking of wine dates back to 5000 B.C. Throughout history it has evoked strong contradictory attitudes and feelings. Some view it as a gift from God and others as the work of the devil. In the earliest days, wine was associated with religion. The feeling of intoxication was often likened to a religious state that allowed drinkers to escape their daily concerns and come closer to the gods. For centuries, wine has been part of the daily diet in many parts of Europe. It has also been closely linked to health. In the nineteenth century, wine was used as a general tonic and prescribed by physicians for a variety of ailments. On the other side has been recognition of the health dangers of excessive drinking. The anti-alcohol movements of the last century especially raised serious doubts about the medicinal benefits of wine.[4]

We can find an abundance of research supporting both the medical benefits of moderate drinking and the damage caused by excessive drinking. In the United States the drinking of wine has primarily been viewed as a recreational activity. Today there is a movement to bring wine back to the table as part of our daily nutrition, as it is in Europe.

Wine can be an integral part of your California Wine Country Diet program if you consume it with conscious indulgence. Recommendations for moderate drinking are one glass a day (5 ounces) for women and two glasses a day (10 ounces) for men. For most wine drinkers, keeping to these limits requires conscious restraint.

The Health Benefits of Alcohol

The American interest in wine was always strong in certain segments of society, but overall its attraction soared following the airing of CBS's "60 Minutes" program *The French Paradox*, in 1991. The show featured French researcher Serge Renaud, who discussed a study that showed that despite their passion for fatty foods, such as butter and cheese, both French men and women have very low rates of coronary heart disease. Researchers attributed this low rate to the French penchant for drinking red wine on a regular basis. It was discovered that red wine in particular, but to some extent also white wine, contains resveratrol, a natural antioxidant that is synthesized in grape skins. Resveratrol has been scientifically shown to lower bad LDL cholesterol while elevating good HDL levels. HDL cholesterol helps clear arterial walls of harmful deposits.[5] Other research has explored the possible anti-aging benefits of resveratrol.

Moderate drinkers also have been found to enjoy better health, suffer fewer heart attacks, and live longer than abstainers or heavy drinkers. Recent studies indicate that the cardiovascular benefit of red wine appears to come from the ethanol found in alcohol, which has a positive effect on the lining of blood vessels. An internationally recognized authority on the health benefits of wine, Dr. Eric Rimm, of the Harvard School of Public Health, says, "Consuming alcohol in moderation either decreases the risk or has no effect on most of the major causes of death in the U.S. Of course, drinking heavily increases the risk of illness and premature death. Moderation is the key."[6]

Alcohol and Weight

As with all other aspects of alcohol, it is possible to find contradictory opinions about the relationship between weight and alcohol. Many diets advocate not drinking at all if you desire to lose weight. Their objections fall into three main areas: that alcohol contains empty calories; that it increases appetite and, consequently, contributes to overeating; and that it slows down metabolism. While the empty-calorie argument may be true for distilled liquor, wine has the same number of calories and nutritional content as grape juice.

The argument that alcohol can lead to overeating by weakening restraint has some validity. One of the most appealing attributes of wine is that it enhances the enjoyment of food, which can cause us to eat more. From a health perspective, this relaxation at the end of a stressful day can be a positive thing. But the delightful feeling one has after a glass of fine wine can make thoughts of weight loss fly out the window, so that we lose our resolve to follow our better judgment about food choices and portions.

As for the relationship between alcohol and metabolism, this is still the subject of vigorous debate. On the positive side is a study by the American Cancer Society of nearly 80,000 healthy adults over a ten-year period that found that alcohol consumption was not associated with gains in body mass index (BMI) for men or women. What is more, wine was the only beverage in the study not associated with a gain of waist circumference in women.[7]

Only you are in a position to evaluate the benefits of alcohol in your weight-loss program and in your life. While the recommendations are for daily consumption of one or two glasses, you may not find it beneficial to drink even a moderate amount of wine or alcohol every day. Or, you may find that you have to alter your choice as you get further into the program.

For example, if you hit a weight-loss plateau, you may want to try decreasing your alcohol consumption to see if this helps get your weight loss moving again. In addition, alcohol consumption has a way of creeping up as we begin to tolerate greater amounts. This tolerance can be readjusted by taking three days off from wine periodically, as you will for the first three days of the food plan. As with all the other aspects of the California Wine Country Diet program, listen to your body and allow it to guide you.

Appreciating Wine

Whether you are new to wine or it is an integral part of your life, including wine in your food plan as a conscious indulgence can be part of making this program an adventure and adding variety to your culinary experience. The appreciation of wine is no longer the province of an elite segment of society. There has never been such variety and abundance of good wine at reasonable prices. If you are just beginning to explore the world of wine, you might want to consult the books on wine listed in the "Suggested Reading and Resources" section at the back of this book. These books will provide you with the basic information to get started learning about and appreciating wine.

But no matter how many books you read, it is the experience of tasting wine that will give you confidence and develop your palate. In order not to be overwhelmed by the profusion of wines on the market, select a particular area in which you wish to be educated. For instance, you might want to explore the wines of a particular winery or a particular varietal from different wineries. You could join a wine club or go on a tasting tour. Your local wine shop may offer tastings or classes.

To begin your education, let us start with the three S's of wine tasting: "Swirl, Sniff, and Sip."

Swirl

In order to fully appreciate wine, it is important to serve it in a decent-size wine glass. The best choice for both red and white wine is a tulip-shaped bowl with a long slender stem, using a larger glass for reds. For sparkling wines, you will need flutes that are tall and thin, which keeps the bubbles moving.

Fill your glass one-third full and have a good look at it against a white background, or hold it up to the sunlight. Notice the color. A lighter color indicates a softer bouquet, or smell and taste. Now swirl the glass in a steady motion, which will release the wine's aromas as it is exposed to air.

Sniff

Hold the glass up to your nose and slowly inhale the wine's aroma. Your first impressions will be the most vivid. While an experienced wine drinker may be able to tell from one sniff exactly where the wine originated, a beginner should start by trying to identify aromas in terms of flavors that are familiar. Does it smell like peach or cocoa or pineapple? Don't worry about being "right." Everyone has his or her own flavor references. Just enjoy the process. Since our sense of smell is directly connected to our sense of taste, these aromatic impressions will enhance the next step of tasting the wine.

Sip

The third step is sipping or tasting. After enjoying the wine's aroma, take a small sip of the wine and roll it around in your mouth. The goal is to allow the wine to reach every part of your tongue. Suck in some air through your lips to open the flavors. Finally, swallow (or spit the wine out if you have many more wines to taste). What is your impression of the wine? Is it sweet or dry? Does it feel heavy or light in your mouth? Does it seem balanced? What flavors are you experiencing? Sweetness will be tasted at the tip of your tongue, saltiness a little further back, acidity or sourness on the sides, peppery at the front, and bitterness at the very back.[8]

Pairing Food and Wine

Choosing the right wine for the meal is another area that causes many people anxiety, especially when they are looking at a long wine list at a restaurant. Once again, experience is the key, and you have to start somewhere. So, don't make yourself a nervous wreck. Anticipate the adventure and also educate yourself. The art of pairing is to choose wine and food that complement each other and do not overwhelm or detract from each other. Most of the restaurant recipes in Chapter 12 include wine suggestions from the chefs. This is an excellent place to increase your understanding of food and wine pairing. Let's look at some general guidelines for pairing food with California wines.[9, 10, 11, 12]

- Forget the old rule you probably grew up with that white wine goes with white meat and red wine with red meat. Be creative.
- Pairing is about finding wine and food that complement each other in a way that increases the enjoyment of both. Neither should overpower the other.
- When wine is served in courses, start with a dry wine before a sweet one, white before red, young before old, and simple before complex.
- When looking for a wine to pair, keep in mind the ingredients of the meal, how the food was prepared and cooked (grilled, steamed, etc.), the herbs and spices used, and any sauces or condiments. Each of these aspects of the meal may affect your wine choice.
- Look to pair a delicate wine with delicate flavors, medium-bodied wines with medium-weight or stronger flavors, and full-bodied or complex wines that can hold their own with intensely flavored foods.
- Highly seasoned, spicy, salty, and smoked flavors are best paired with light, fruity wines such as Gewurztraminer, Riesling, and Pinot Noir.
- Rich and fatty foods such as lamb, beef, cheese, and duck work well with full-bodied Chardonnay, Cabernet Sauvignon, Merlot, Zinfandel, and Syrah.
- With sweet foods you want to be sure that the sweetness of the

dish is less sweet than the sweetness of the wine. Wines with sweetness include Johannisberg Reisling, Gewurztraminer, and White Zinfandel.

- High acid foods such as tomatoes, citrus fruits, and goat cheese go best with acidic wines such as Sauvignon Blanc, certain styles of Chardonnay, Zinfandel, Pinot Noir, and Sangiovese.

- When cooking with wine, be sure to use a good quality wine. Using this same wine to drink, paired with your dinner, is a sensible choice.

These suggestions and recommendations, of course, only touch the tip of the iceberg of the complex subject of wine and food pairing.

Many wineries list pairing suggestions for their wines. Restaurants are increasingly making suggestions for pairings on their menus. You can learn a great deal by talking to the wine waiter or sommelier. Above all, remember that this exploration is for your enjoyment. While there may be a few "perfect pairings," for the most part you are simply looking for the combination that pleases you.

Conscious Indulgence with Wine

Just as you were getting into the exciting world of wine exploration, here I am bringing up conscious indulgence. Learning the subtleties of wine and the complexities of pairing can actually help you with being more conscious about the wine you drink.

Following the USDA Dietary Guidelines of five ounces a day for women and ten ounces a day for men is not always easy for those who love wine. Therefore, focusing on the taste of the wine you do drink will help you get the most pleasure from it. Drinking moderately is not only good for your health but may encourage you to investigate some more expensive wines, since you will be drinking only one or two glasses a day. Let us look at ways to satisfy your love of wine while remaining conscious of your indulgence in this pleasure:

- When at home, measure out 2.5 ounces and 5 ounces of wine in your favorite wine glasses. If these glasses have designs on them, use the designs as fill-to guides, so you can easily know how much to pour the next time.

- While wine is meant to be enjoyed with food, you can decide which course you most want to have your wine with. Perhaps it will be with an appetizer as you make dinner. Or maybe you want to save your wine to have with a special dessert. You can also divide your wine servings between courses.

- When at a wine tasting, learn the art of spitting. Or just sip a small amount and pour the rest of the wine in your glass into one of the buckets usually supplied for this. Getting rid of wonderful wine is a hard habit to acquire, but it is the only way to keep within your alcohol guidelines in situations where you will be tasting many different wines.

- Do not forget to subtract the calories of your wine from your daily pleasure food calories. White wine has 100 calories and red wine 106 calories per five-ounce serving.

- Few of us are content to nurse five ounces of wine over a lengthy period of time, say from before dinner through the serving of dessert. Therefore, it is helpful to have nonalcoholic beverages conveniently available that you can enjoy before, during, or after your wine. We will look more closely at this important tip now.

The Pleasure of Non-Alcoholic Beverages

When they hear the title of this book, most people ask me one of two questions: "Does this mean I can drink all the wine I want and still lose weight?" And, "Do I have to drink wine to be on this diet?" The answer to both questions is "No."

While most of our nutritional focus in the California Wine Country Diet program has been on food, beverages do play a key role in any weight-management program. They are often overlooked sources of calories and so can be the main cause of weight gain. The beverages we choose to drink can also affect the state of our health. For example, between the late 1970s and the late 1990s, soft-drink consumption in the United States by adults rose 61 percent and more than doubled for children. A study of more than 90,000 young and middle-aged women published in the *Jour-*

nal of the American Medical Association[13] suggests that a woman who consumes just one can of a soft drink a day is 83 percent more likely to acquire diabetes than a woman who has less than one such beverage a month. Women drinking one or more cans of soda a day during the time period of the study gained an average of twenty pounds, whereas those who drank at the lower level of consumption gained just three pounds.

Drinking fruit juice is certainly healthier than drinking sodas, but just as with wine, attention must be given to the calories consumed. Drinking orange juice is not nearly as filling as eating an orange.

Our number-one choice of a beverage to drink should be water. The conventional wisdom has been to drink eight ten-ounce glasses of water a day. Water has no calories. We need it, and on a hot day after exercising there is nothing we would rather drink. On the other hand, when you are out for a special meal at a nice restaurant and everyone else is enjoying his or her second glass of wine, having a glass of water does not seem satisfying. That is why you have to begin to expand your beverage choices. You do not have to choose between only wine or water. You could drink sparkling or soda water with a slice of lemon or lime, or any number of other choices.

Alice Waters, the founder of Chez Panisse restaurant, says that she has been researching nonalcoholic beverages that "not only enhance the food but can be as ritualistic as sharing a bottle of wine at the table." She looks for beverages that are not too sweet such as a tea-like drink called *tisane* that is made by plunging freshly picked herbs such as mint and chamomile into boiling water. At the French Laundry restaurant in Yountville, California, Chef Thomas Keller has given his wine and beverage chef, Paul Roberts, the mission to find the perfect nonalcoholic beverage to go with each course of the meal for those customers who do not drink alcohol or who are limiting their consumption. Roberts has paired pasta with a small foaming glass of Clover Stornetta whole milk, lobster fricassee with Meyer Lemon GuS soda, and Coho salmon roe sprinkled over a buttery porridge with a glass of chilled chamomile tea.[14] Here are some ideas for what you can do at home to enjoy the pleasures of beverages other wine.

As Alice Waters points out, part of the pleasure of wine is the sense of ritual around it. You can make other beverages feel special by putting them in wine glasses or champagne flutes. Place a slice of lemon, lime, or orange at the rim of the glass. Decorate the glass with a sprig of mint or sip it through a special straw.

Have a variety of bottled water chilled, and bring a bottle to the table to pour when you have had your limit of wine.

Take sparkling water or club soda and place it in a flute with one or two tablespoons of fruit juice. You can enjoy the taste of the juice and the bubbles with few added calories.

Explore the wonderful world of tea. There are hundreds of different teas available, from peppermint to raspberry to hazelnut. Drinking tea can energize you or calm you down depending on the variety. Both green and black teas contain many of the same antioxidants found in wine, many that have been studied for their tumor regression properties and other anticancer activities.[15] Other health benefits attributed to drinking tea include a lower risk of heart disease, lower blood pressure, lower cholesterol, and more stable blood sugar levels.[16]

The same teas you enjoy hot can be delicious iced. Iced tea makers simplify this process so that you always have some iced tea ready in the refrigerator. This is an excellent alternative to sodas for the whole family. Experiment with pairing different teas with food. Unless you add sugar, this is a healthy beverage that adds no calories.

By now you should have greatly expanded your conception of pleasure foods. Make selecting your pleasure foods each day an enjoyable experience by adding variety and by consciously indulging yourself. In Chapter 12, you will be exploring a different aspect of wine and pleasure by "visiting" the California wine country and learning the secrets of some of its chefs' most delectable and healthful recipes.

Chapter 12
California Wine Country Restaurant Recipes

"What we are looking for with food and all we do in the kitchen is epiphany...[When food] is so overwhelming and so joyous you fall to the ground...You speak in tongues... because you are so overwhelmed with the [taste]."

— *John Ash*

We are about to embark upon a great culinary adventure. In this chapter we'll have the opportunity to visit California's different wine-growing areas and individual restaurants in these areas that serve wine country cuisine. Since space allows only a sampling of the wonderful recipes from some of the best restaurants in the wine country, I have given Web site addresses to help you explore further.

Gathering these recipes has given me a whole new appreciation of chefs and what goes into making the delicious dishes they prepare for us. The recipes included will give you the chance to experiment with California wine country cuisine in the comfort of your own home. One of the greatest pleasures for me in working on this book was preparing these recipes. While some were more challenging than others for a novice cook such as myself, I can honestly say that every single recipe I prepared was sumptuous.

Twelve recipes, four each week, have been integrated into the Daily Meal Plans of your first three weeks on the California Wine Country Diet. Then, when these three weeks are over, you can use the recipes you've tried or experiment with others. Having this variety is an important key in keeping you from the diet doldrums. Don't be intimidated by some of the exotic-sounding ingredients, for they may open a whole new world of pleasure to you.

Most of the recipes include suggested wine pairings. While it is not possible to list individual wineries, you will also be given resources for finding wineries in each of the California wine-growing areas. California is the leading wine-producing state in the United States. Two out of every three bottles of domestic wine sold in this country comes from California. Vineyards are situated across the state from the coast to the inland valleys to the mountain foothills. Let's begin with the northern most wine-growing region, Humboldt County.

Humboldt County

Humboldt Online Directory: www.humboldt.info

Far better known for redwood trees than vineyards, Humboldt County is a beautiful and relaxing place to begin or end any trip to California. After a day exploring Humboldt Redwoods State Park, which has the largest remaining stand of virgin redwoods in the world, head for the Benbow Inn, listed on the National Register of Historic Places, in Garberville. First opening its doors in 1926, the inn was designed for the Benbow family by noted architect Albert Farr. It became a favorite get-away for Hollywood stars such as Spencer Tracy, Clark Gable, and Alan Ladd, as well as dignitaries like Eleanor Roosevelt and Herbert Hoover. The inn has maintained its elegant hospitality and peaceful atmosphere to this day. Settling back into the rich velvet chairs in front of a crackling fire for afternoon tea, it is easy to imagine that you are at a country estate in England.

The restaurant at the Benbow Inn serves breakfast and dinner, also lunch during the summer. Chef Marci Bame trained at the California Culinary Academy. She has worked at the Robert Mondavi Winery, the Grille at the Depot in Park City, Utah, Left at Albuquerque in San Francisco, and Roxanne's in Marin County. The restaurant uses locally grown produce, some from its own gardens, and features local Humboldt County wines.

Benbow Inn
445 Lake Benbow Drive, Garberville, CA 95542
(707) 923-2124 or (800) 355-3301
www.benbowinn.com

Recipes from the Benbow Inn Restaurant

by Executive Chef Marci Bame

Grilled Wild Salmon with Dill and Yogurt Mashed Potatoes and Whole-Grain Mustard Vinaigrette

Serves 4

Grilled Wild Salmon

4 4-ounce portions Pacific wild salmon, skin on
Salt and pepper to taste
Nonstick cooking spray

To grill the salmon, spray the fish with a nonstick cooking spray and season with kosher salt and freshly ground black pepper.
Nutrition pyramid servings: 4 protein

Dill and Yogurt Mashed Potatoes

1½ pounds russet potatoes, peeled and cut into quarters
1/3 cup plain fat-free yogurt
2 tablespoons fresh dill
½ teaspoon kosher salt
2 to 4 tablespoons fat-free milk

Cut the potatoes into large cubes and boil in a pot of water until soft. Strain out the water and mash the potatoes with a potato masher. Add the rest of the ingredients and serve.
Nutrition pyramid servings: 2 grain

Whole-Grain Mustard Vinaigrette

Makes ¾ cup, 8 servings

1 garlic clove
4 tablespoons lemon juice
1 lemon zested
1½ tablespoons whole grained mustard
½ cup virgin olive oil
½ cup fresh chives, chopped
Salt and pepper to taste

Put the garlic and a pinch of salt into a bowl, crush together, then stir in the lemon zest and juice. Add the mustard and mix until smooth.

Slowly pour the oil into the bowl, whisking continually until emulsified. Add chives and season with the black pepper. Serve on potatoes and salmon.

Nutrition pyramid servings: 1 oil

Chef's wine suggestion: Sauvignon Blanc or un-oaked Chardonnay with a citrus finish.

This is a wonderful way to cook salmon without adding any extra calories. It is an easy dish for any night of the week. The only added fat is in the vinaigrette, which makes it easy to control the amount you use. You might want to try the potatoes and vinaigrette with another fish or chicken dish when salmon is out of season.

Mendocino County—Inland

www.goMendo.com

Traveling south from Humboldt County on Highway 101 you will arrive in another beautiful rural county, Mendocino. This sparsely populated county covers over 3,500 square miles, from the breathtaking splendor of the coast to vineyard-covered hills, redwood forests, and rugged mountains. With a population of 15,000, Ukiah is the seat of county government and the largest town. It is the hub of Mendocino wine country, offering wineries and tasting rooms nearby, with short drives to Redwood Valley, Hopland, and Anderson Valley.

While there have been wine grapes growing here since the 1850s, Mendocino County wines were relatively unknown—compared to Napa and Sonoma—until the 1970s. Parducci Wine Cellars and Fetzer Vineyards led the way to national and worldwide distinction. Combining a strong regional emphasis on organic grape-growing with attention to the different varietals that can be grown in Mendocino's many microclimates is ushering in a new era in Mendocino's wine industry.

In Ukiah's historic downtown you will find Patrona Bistro and Wine Bar, which exemplifies the principles of California wine country cuisine. Italian and Spanish influences inspire local and sustainably produced ingredients. The wine list includes wine from each of Mendocino's fifty-eight wineries as well as other California and European wines. Chefs and co-owners Bridget Harrington and Craig Strattman explain how they chose the name of their restaurant: "As chefs we are extremely honored to have as our medium these amazing products we call food that are produced not by humans but by the earth herself. … At our restaurant, we have adopted *Patrona* as the symbol for this great force of nature and spirit that guides us."

Patrona Bistro and Wine Bar
130 W. Standley Street
Ukiah, CA 95482
(707) 462-9181
www.patronarestaurant.com

Recipes from Patrona Bistro and Wine Bar

by Bridget Harrington, Chef and Owner

Cioppino

Serves 6–8
¼ cup extra-virgin olive oil
2 cups chopped onion
6–8 large cloves of garlic, minced

2 28-ounce cans crushed tomatoes (Muir Glen is best)
2 cups hearty red wine
1 large whole bay leaf
1–2 teaspoons dried oregano or 1 tablespoon fresh
1–2 teaspoons dried basil or 1 tablespoon fresh
4 cups fish stock (use shrimp shells and fish bones)
½–1 cup dry sherry
1 pound firm white fish (halibut, haddock, cod…), cut into cubes
1 pound peeled and deveined medium shrimp, tail off
Clams, mussels, cockles, scallops, as you wish
6 crab claws (also optional)
Salt and pepper to taste
Tapatío or Tabasco sauce to taste

Heat oil in a large non-reactive pot over medium-high heat. When oil is hot, add onions and cook, stirring often until translucent. Add garlic and cook until fragrant, about 1 minute. Add wine and reduce until onions are lightly coated with wine "syrup." Add tomatoes, herbs, and fish stock, and cook over medium-low heat for about 2 hours.

While this cooks, prepare your fish. If you are using bivalves, soak them in cold saltwater for 20 minutes. Rinse and repeat. Take any beards off the mussels.

One half-hour before eating, add sherry, salt, pepper and hot sauce.

Ten minutes before eating, adjust flavors again and add fish. Bivalves should go in first. Wait a couple of minutes and add the fish. The shrimp should be added right at the end as they will take less than a minute to cook.

To garnish, place a crab claw on top with a sprig of fresh herbs.

Serve with crusty bread, olives, green salad.

Nutrition pyramid servings: 4 meat, 1.5 vegetable, 2 oil (omit if using spray instead of olive oil)

Chef's wine suggestion: Sangiovese or Zinfandel.

Make this amazing cioppino on an evening when you have leisurely time to prepare it. It makes a wonderful meal for family or entertaining. If the fish is out of season it is still delicious with frozen clams, mussels, shrimp and white fish.

Zinfandel Braised Pot Roast

Serves 18
1 4-pound beef chuck roast (organic preferred)
3 teaspoons sea salt
2 teaspoons freshly cracked ground pepper
2 tablespoons fragrant Spanish paprika
2 tablespoons chopped fresh rosemary
½ cup all-purpose flour
¼ cup olive oil
½ pound pancetta, diced
2 yellow onions, peeled and cut lengthwise into 8 pieces
4 ribs of celery, diced
2 carrots, cut into 2-inch chunks
1 tablespoon minced garlic
1 bay leaf
1 28-ounce can whole tomatoes (Muir Glen preferred)
1 cup good-quality beef stock
3 cups Zinfandel wine (Fetzer preferred!)
Salt and pepper to taste

Preheat oven to 350 degrees. In a small bowl, mix salt, pepper, paprika, and rosemary. Rub mixture well into meat and let sit for at least 2 hours. Bring meat to room temperature and coat with a little olive oil and a dusting of flour. Heat a Dutch oven to high and brown the meat on all sides. This should take 7 to 10 minutes.

Remove meat to a platter and add the pancetta, onions, celery, and carrots to the Dutch oven. Cook until vegetables are beginning to brown. Drain off the fat, add the meat back to the Dutch oven, and add garlic, bay leaf, tomatoes (crush them up with your hands), beef stock, and wine. Cook covered for about 2 hours then check for doneness. Cooking time will vary depending on temperature of meat after searing, the Dutch oven material, and your oven. It is done when a knife slices very easily through it. You be the judge. You may have to let these cook for up to 4 or 5 hours. When you do feel it is done, drain off cooking liquid, skim off the fat and reduce to sauce consistency.

The roast must rest for at least 30 minutes before serving, but is even better if kept for serving the next day. Simply slice the roast and serve with sauce and vegetables. Creamy polenta or potatoes are always a nice accompaniment to this rustic dish.

Nutrition pyramid servings: 4 meat, .75 vegetable, .5 oil

Chef's wine suggestion: A nice glass of Zinfandel

Home cook Ellen Holmes, who has cooked many pot roasts in her day, raves about this recipe. She says that for those who have the time and patience to cook it, "It is so worth the wait."

South of Ukiah lies the small town of Hopland and the Fetzer Vineyards Valley Oak Ranch. In the 1980s, the Fetzer family and then president Paul Dolan began to turn the ranch into a world-class food and wine education center. At the center of Valley Oaks Ranch is the five-acre organic garden that was reproduced by Garden Director Kate Frey at the Chelsea Flower Show in London, winning a Silver medal in 2003 and a Gold in 2005 from the Royal Horticultural Society. Visitors are invited to taste the edible plants as they stroll in the gardens, which provide fresh herbs, vegetables, and fruits for Fetzer Vineyards Café.

Fetzer was the first major winery to embrace organic wine grape-growing techniques and is one of the largest to do so in the world. Brown-Forman, a Kentucky-based liquor company, bought Fetzer Vineyards from the Fetzer family and has continued their commitment to organic growing and sustainable business practices.

Valley Oaks Ranch Food and Beverage Director Bridget Harrington says that her first introduction to real food came during her senior year at the University of San Francisco, when she traveled to study in Italy. After returning to graduate school, to pay her tuition, Bridget began cooking for caterers (including her now husband and co-owner of Patrona, Craig Strattman). By 1988, she was catering herself and acquired Fetzer Vineyards as a client in 1995. Joining the winery as executive chef in 1999, she was excited and honored to work for John Ash, who served for many years as the culinary director of Fetzer Vineyards. During her tenure at Fetzer, Bridget initiated an educational program for Hopland and Ukiah children to learn about food—and in which they make their own lunch. She is also working with the Ukiah and Sonoma County school districts to overhaul their school nutrition programs.

Fetzer Valley Oaks Ranch
13601 Eastside Road
Hopland, CA 95449
(800) 846-8637
www.Fetzer.com

Recipes from Fetzer Vineyards Café at Valley Oaks Ranch

by Food and Beverage Director Bridget Harrington

Mediterranean Chicken

Serves 8–16

½ cup capers

1/3 cup minced garlic

1 tablespoon each oregano, basil, thyme, and bay

½ cup olive oil

½ cup red wine vinegar

Salt and pepper

2 whole chickens cut up into 8 pieces each

8 ounces of dry white wine

1/3 cup brown sugar

1 cup dried apricots

1½ cups small green olives, pitted

Mix first 6 ingredients together in a bowl and pour over chickens. Marinate overnight. Place skin side up in 1 or 2 roasting pans with the marinade. Pour dry white wine over the chicken and sprinkle with brown sugar. Bake at 350 degrees for about 1 hour or until chicken is done. Remove chicken skin before serving to reduce fat content.

Pour sauce remaining in pan into a bowl, skim off fat, and reduce over high heat until it is a nice sauce consistency. Place chicken on a warm platter, spoon apricots and olives on top, and pour sauce over all.

Serve with couscous.

Nutrition pyramid servings: 3–4 protein, .25 fruit, 1.5 oil
(One serving = 3 to 4 ounces of chicken, ½ cup sauce)

This delicious recipe is one that you can easily make ahead of time for either your family or guests. The ingredients are available all year around. For a smaller amount simply use one chicken and cut all the other ingredients in half.

Thai Spring Rolls with Spicy Peanut Dipping Sauce

Thai Spring Rolls
Rice-paper wrappers
Assorted raw vegetables:
   carrot
   daikon
   Napa cabbage
   red pepper
   cucumber
   mung bean sprouts
   snow peas
   pickled ginger
   Thai basil (cut in thin strips, also known as chiffonade)

All vegetables should be thinly julienned (cut in match-stick-like strips). Using various colors makes an eye-appealing dish.

Place a clean, dry towel (cotton or linen) on your counter. In a bowl of tepid water place 1 rice wrapper and soak until soft (30 seconds to 1 minute). Arrange vegetables, basil, and ginger in center and roll up like a burrito; continue until you have the quantity you want. When ready to serve, slice in half on diagonal and serve with dipping sauce. May be kept wrapped in plastic, for a couple of hours.

*Nutrition pyramid serving*s: 1 roll = .5 grain, 1 vegetable

Spicy Peanut Dipping Sauce
¼ cup finely chopped cilantro
¼ cup finely chopped toasted peanuts
2/3 cup fish sauce
2/3 cup rice wine vinegar
1 teaspoon orange zest
1 teaspoon minced hot red dried pepper, seeded
1 tablespoon minced garlic
5 tablespoons sugar

Combine ingredients and let flavors meld at least 1 hour.
Nutrition pyramid servings: 2 tablespoons = free food

Chef's suggested wine: Serve with a wine that has a little residual sugar such as Gewurztraminer or Riesling.

Fish sauce is popular throughout Southeast Asia. It is a strongly flavored mixture based on liquid from salted, fermented fish and is used for flavoring in much the same way that soy sauce is. It can be found in Asian markets and in the Asian section of your supermarket. The Thai Spring Rolls are an easy and unique way to prepare fresh vegetables. You might want to let everyone prepare their own rolls so they get exactly the vegetables they want.

Mendocino Coast
It's time now to leave inland Mendocino County and head for the coast. When those from other areas hear the word *Mendocino* they most often think of the town of Mendocino. This historic town that boasts of

having no supermarkets, fast food restaurants, or motels is located on the headlands above the Pacific Ocean. No wonder people from all over the world come to rest and enjoy a slower pace of life. Mornings can be spent exploring the beauty of nature, then stopping for lunch at one of the many fine restaurants in town or nearby along the coast. Afterwards there are shops, art galleries, and museums to visit. Throughout the year music, art, food, and wine events provide entertainment for visitors.

Two miles south of Mendocino is the village of Little River and beautiful Van Damme State Park. The grand Victorian house that eventually became the Little River Inn was built as a family home in the 1850s by Silas Coombs, a lumberman from Maine.

In 1939 Coombs' daughter Cora and her husband, Ole Herville, bought the home from her parents and opened the Little River Inn. The delicious home cooking, family hospitality, and spectacular ocean views have been bringing visitors back to the inn for over sixty years. Food is served in both Ole's Whale Watch Bar and the Garden-View Dining Room.

Little River Inn's executive chef, Silver Canul, grew up in the Yucatan in Mexico, where at age eight he began to help cook for his nine brothers and sisters. Arriving in California in 1985, his first jobs were picking peas and milking cows. As a prep cook at the Heritage House, he was noticed by renowned chef Eric Lenard, who personally trained him. He has supplemented his training with studies at the Culinary Academy of America in Napa. In 1995, he became executive chef of the Little River Inn where he combines traditional California cuisine with a cooking style that reflects the distinctive flavors of his Mayan heritage.

Little River Inn
Little River, CA 95456
www.littleriverinn.com
888-466-5683 or 707-937-5942

Recipes from the Little River Inn
by Chef Silver Canul

Grilled Eggplant and Portabello Mushrooms with Tomato and Sweet Pepper Sauce

Serves 4

2 large eggplants
3 tablespoons extra-virgin olive oil
5 portabello mushrooms
2 tablespoons chopped shallots
2 tablespoons chopped garlic
½ white onion, sliced
2 tomatoes, diced
½ red sweet pepper, sliced
½ gold sweet pepper, sliced
½ cup tomato juice
3 tablespoons chopped fresh basil
1 tablespoon butter (optional)
6 ounces part-skim mozzarella cheese

Slice each eggplant lengthwise into 4 slices. Each slice should be about a half-inch thick. Brush with olive oil and sprinkle with salt and pepper. Charbroil the eggplant slices quickly on high heat until the slices are nice and golden, with grill marks, about 2½ minutes each side. (If you don't have a grill or a grill pan, you can sauté the eggplant in olive oil.) Set aside and let cool.

Brush the mushrooms with olive oil, sprinkle with salt and pepper, and grill in the same manner. Set aside and let cool.

Heat the remaining olive oil in a saucepan, and quickly cook the shallots and garlic over high heat, about 1 minute. Stir in the rest of the vegetables and cook over medium heat for about 8 minutes. Stir in the tomato juice, and continue cooking over low heat until the vegetables are soft, about 10 minutes. Remove from heat and stir in the basil, and butter if desired. Set the mixture aside to cool. (If you are in a hurry, spread it on a baking sheet to cool it down faster.) It's important to have all the ingredients at the same temperature when you assemble them for baking.

Slice the cooked portabello mushrooms at an angle. Place 4 eggplant slices on a baking sheet, over a light dab of butter or oil to prevent sticking. Top each slice with a good tablespoon of sauce, and arrange some portabello slices over the sauce. Top each with a slice of mozzarella cheese, then with another slice of eggplant.

Bake for about 8 minutes at 375 degrees. Serve with a small amount of sauce on each plate.

© 2000 SILVER CANUL

Nutrition pyramid servings: 5 vegetable, 2 oil, 1 dairy
Chef's wine suggestion: Navarro Mendocino Pinot Noir.

Everyone who has tried this dish has loved it. Even if you think you don't like eggplant, try it. The recipe is easy enough for a weeknight and special enough for entertaining. To cut oil, use oil spray instead of brushing oil on the vegetables.

Halibut with Panko Chips and Pecans with Tropical Mango Salsa

Serves 4

Halibut with Panko Chips and Pecans
2 pounds halibut filets (no bones)
¼ cup chopped pecans
¼ cup panko chips (Japanese breadcrumbs)
1 egg
1 cup fat-free evaporated milk
Olive oil & butter for sautéing

Apportion about 8 ounces of halibut per person. Combine the pecans and panko chips, and do the same with the egg and the milk.

Dip the halibut in the egg wash, shake off the excess, and place into the pecan-chip mixture, pressing gently with your hands.

Heat olive oil and butter in a sauté pan, and cook the halibut for 3 minutes on each side.

Garnish with mango salsa, and serve with fresh asparagus or another vegetable of your choice.

Nutrition pyramid servings: 4 mcat, 23 pleasure food calories; if butter and oil are used add 22 pleasure food calories.

Tropical Mango Salsa
Makes 1 quart

2 oranges
8 mangoes, peeled and diced
3 fresh Roma tomatoes, peeled and diced
½ bunch fresh cilantro, chopped
½ red onion, finely chopped
½ cantaloupe, finely diced
Salt to taste
½ teaspoon cayenne pepper
Juice of 1 lime

Peel the oranges, making sure to remove all of the bitter-tasting white pithy part. Remove the segments by slicing between each membrane with a sharp knife. Then squeeze the juice into a large bowl.

Mix in the remaining ingredients, and chill until ready to serve.

Nutrition pyramid servings: ¼ cup = 1.5 fruit

Chef's wine suggestion: Husch Special Reserve Mendocino Charodonnay.

For the salsa, you can save time by buying a jar of prepared mangos. If you can't find panko chips use plain breadcrumbs. If halibut is not in season, this recipe works well with cod. The original recipe called for half and half which we replaced with fat-free evaporated milk.

Grilled Mexican White Prawns with a Tomato, Habañero Chile and Mushroom Sauce

Serves 4 as an appetizer

3 vine-ripened tomatoes

1 habañero chile
1 shallot, minced
2 cloves garlic, chopped
1 cup sliced shiitake mushrooms
1 teaspoon unsalted butter
¼ teaspoon lemon juice
Pinch of brown sugar
Salt and pepper to taste
1 tablespoon basil chiffonade (leaves rolled and thinly sliced)
12 large Mexican prawns
Canola oil for basting

Grill the tomatoes for about 8 minutes. Grill the habañero for about 4 minutes.

Sauté the garlic and shallot for about 1 minute. Add the mushrooms and cook for about 6 minutes. Remove from heat; mix in the grilled tomatoes and half of the habañero. Put the pan back over medium heat and add the butter, lemon juice, sugar, and salt and pepper. Finish with the basil.

Meanwhile, you can be grilling the prawns, seasoned to taste with salt and pepper, basting with the canola oil. Grill for about 6 minutes. Place 3 prawns on each plate, top with a few spoonsful of sauce, and enjoy!

© 2001 SILVER CANUL

Nutrition pyramid servings: 3 prawns = .75 meat, 2 vegetable, .5 oil

Chef's wine suggestion: Swanson Pinot Grigio

Those who enjoy a spicy dish will love these prawns. The habañero chile makes this a hot dish. Use an olive oil spray in the pan for the sauté. For a main dish serve 6 prawns each with rice and grilled vegetables.

Dungeness Crab Cakes

Serves 8 as an appetizer or 4 as a dinner entree

1½ pounds cooked Dungeness crabmeat
2 tablespoons chopped onions

2 tablespoons chopped celery

2 tablespoons chopped sweet peppers

2 tablespoons Dijon mustard

2 tablespoons mayonnaise (fat-free)

1 tablespoon chopped fresh basil

1 tablespoon chopped cilantro

1 ½ tablespoons lime juice

½ teaspoon Tabasco sauce

½ cup breadcrumbs, plus extra for coating cakes

2 or 3 tablespoons olive oil

In a large bowl, mix together all the ingredients except the olive oil. The mixture should be nice and thick, but not too thick. If it is too loose, add more breadcrumbs. Make 8 equal-sized balls and then pat each ball into a cake-like shape. Roll the cakes in breadcrumbs and set aside.

Preheat a large pan and add the olive oil. When it is beginning to smoke, slowly add the cakes. Adjust the heat to medium and sear the cakes for about 2 minutes on each side. Serve with slices of lime. Accompany the cakes with guacamole and diced tomatoes as an appetizer, or with wild rice and fresh steamed vegetables as a dinner entree.

Nutrition pyramid servings: one patty = .5 grain, 2.5 protein, .75 oil

This is a wonderful crab cake recipe that I am sure you will enjoy. To cut down on the amount of olive oil, use an olive oil spray. Make sure to chop the vegetables finely and to squeeze the excess liquid from the crab and vegetables. While fresh crab is the best, this recipe also works well with canned crab.

Four miles down the Pacific Coast Highway you will arrive at the Albion River Inn, recognized as having one of the finest restaurants on the Mendocino coast. Recipient of praise from regional and national press, as well as magazines such as *Bon Appetit*, *The Wine Spectator*, and *Sunset*, the Albion River Inn has built its culinary reputation on hearty and innovative regional cuisine highlighted by fresh seafood and an award-winning wine and spirits list. Executive Chef Stephen Smith describes his style as "a meeting of Mendocino's bounty and my own very eclectic culinary taste." Chef Smith began his culinary career in the Albion River Inn kitchen and then moved to the Bay Area for further training at the California Culinary Academy. He has worked at renowned Stars Restaurant in San Francisco under Jeremiah Tower and taught at Sacramento's acclaimed Chinois East/West. In 1992, he returned to the inn and became executive chef in 1993 at the age of twenty-six.

Albion River Inn
P.O. Box 100
Albion, CA 95410
800-479-7944 or 707-937-1919
www.albionriverinn.com

Recipes from the Albion River Inn

by Executive Chef Stephen Smith

Pan-Seared King Salmon with Steamed Shellfish in Fennel-Tomato Broth

Serves 4–8

Coconut-Steamed Jasmine Rice
2 cups water
4 ounces unsweetened coconut milk (reduce fat by using fat free evaporated milk)
1 tablespoon granulated sugar
1 tablespoon salt
1 cup jasmine rice

Make the jasmine rice first and leave covered. It will retain its heat until it is served. In a small pan heat the water, salt, sugar, and milk until boiling. Add the rice, and stir until rice simmers. Reduce heat to medium low and cover tightly. Simmer for 20 minutes. Remove from heat.
Nutrition pyramid servings: With coconut milk, 2 grain, 45 pleasure food calories. With fat-free evaporated milk, 2 grain .25 dairy.

Pan-Seared King Salmon with Steamed Shellfish

Serves 8

- 2 ounces olive oil (or use 1 tablespoon olive oil and olive oil spray to reduce fat)
- 8 3-ounce fresh salmon filets
- Salt and pepper
- 16 fresh clams
- 16 fresh mussels
- 4 large prawns
- 2 ounces olive oil
- 1 small fennel bulb, julienne (sliced in match-stick-like pieces)
- 1 small yellow onion, julienned
- 1 tablespoon fresh minced garlic
- 1 large tomato, diced
- 4 ounces white wine
- 16 ounces fish stock (clam juice or chicken stock will work also)
- 2 tablespoons fresh basil, chopped
- 2 tablespoons tomato paste
- 1 carrot, peeled and julienned
- 1 zucchini
- 4 tablespoons fresh basil blended with 2 ounces fat-free sour cream (optional for drizzling on top)

In a large sauté pan, heat 2 ounces olive oil until almost smoking. Season fish with salt and pepper, and cook in pan for 5 minutes on each side. Meanwhile, in a large pot heat 2 ounces olive oil until almost smoking. Add fennel, onion, garlic, and tomato; cook for 5 minutes on medium heat. Add white wine and reduce for 3 minutes. Add stock, fresh basil, and tomato paste, and stir to incorporate. Add mussels, clams, and prawns, and simmer until shellfish is all open—about 5 minutes. Add carrot and zucchini at the last minute. Ladle broth with 4 clams and 4 mussels into serving bowl. Place jasmine rice in middle of bowl. Place salmon on top of rice and prawn on top of salmon with zucchini and carrot for garnish. Drizzle with basil cream if desired.

Nutrition pyramid servings: 4 meat, 1 vegetable, 4 oil (.5 oil if oil spray used). Basil cream garnish = free food

This is a scrumptious seafood dish. Despite the many ingredients, it is relatively easy to make and is another dish you might want to use for entertaining. If out of season, clams, mussels, and prawns are all good frozen. While this dish is traditionally prepared with coconut milk in the jasmine rice, for the purposes of a low-fat diet substitute fat-free evaporated milk.

Peppered Ahi Tuna with Mongolian Barbecue Glaze and Napa Cabbage Salad

Serves 8

Peppered Ahi Tuna

8 3-ounce fresh ahi tuna steaks cut 1 inch thick

2 tablespoons whole black peppercorns (freshly cracked into coarse pieces)

Salt and pepper—sprinkled on fish

Fresh lemon juice—sprinkled on fish

8 teaspoons peanut oil (spray pan then use 1 teaspoon peanut oil per serving of fish)

Prepare fish and let sit for 5 minutes before searing. Heat oil in sauté pan until smoking. Add the seasoned fish and cook on high heat for 1 minute on each side. Pour oil out of pan. Add glaze (see below) and cook fish for 30 seconds more. Remove from pan. Thinly slice and place on Napa Cabbage Salad (see below).

Nutrition pyramid servings: 3 meat, 1 oil

Mongolian Barbecue Glaze

2 ounces mild red chili sauce or ketchup

2 ounces oyster sauce

2 ounces Hoisin sauce

2 ounces rice wine vinegar

1 tablespoon red chili flakes

2 tablespoons brown sugar

1 teaspoon ginger—minced

1 teaspoon garlic—minced

2 ounces peanut oil

Heat oil in small sauce pan. Combine all ingredients and carefully add to oil. Whisk to incorporate. Simmer on medium-low for 5 minutes.
Nutrition pyramid servings: 2 tablespoons = 1.5 oil

Napa Cabbage Salad

2 cups Napa cabbage—thinly sliced

1 cucumber—peeled, seeded, and sliced

1 red bell pepper—julienned

1 red onion—julienned

3 green onions—sliced

2 tablespoons fresh ginger—minced

½ bunch whole cilantro leaves

2 ounces soy sauce

1 ounce rice wine vinegar

½ teaspoon sesame oil

Combine in bowl and let sit 30 minutes. Mix well before serving.
Nutrition pyramid servings: 1 vegetable

Do not let the long list of ingredients discourage you from trying these wonderful recipes. Save some undressed Napa Cabbage Salad for lunch the next day. Enjoy all the Asian ingredients in the Mongolian Barbecue Glaze. You should be able to find them in the Asian section of your supermarket.

Sonoma County

Sonoma County Wineries Association: www.sonomawine.com
Sonoma County Tourism Program: www.sonomacounty.com

Leaving the coast and heading back inland via Route 128 into Sonoma County takes you through the beautiful vineyards of several renowned viticultural areas including Dry Creek, Alexander Valley, and Russian River. Grapes were first planted in Sonoma County by the Franciscian padres in the 1820s. The county is blessed with rich soil and varied climate that stretches from the cool breezes of the Pacific all the way to the San Francisco Bay. Nearly every type of grape can be grown here, from the cool-weather loving Pinot Noir to warm-weather Zinfandel. In addition to the bounty from the Pacific Ocean, 56 percent of Sonoma County is farmland that is devoted to dairy farms, livestock rangeland, fruit orchards, and, of course, vineyards.

The town of Healdsburg is an excellent place from which to explore the wineries of northern Sonoma County. The town is built around a classic town square where you will find an abundance of good food and small shops to explore. Right on the square is the Hotel Healdsburg, a full-service luxury hotel that is the site of acclaimed chef Charlie Palmer's Dry Creek Kitchen. Chef Palmer, who now resides in Healdsburg, is one of the most regarded chefs in America. The author of three books, he has other restaurants in New York, Washington, D.C., Las Vegas, and Los Angeles.

At the Dry Creek Kitchen, he focuses on "highlighting Sonoma County's fresh ingredients with an ever-changing menu" and an all-Sonoma wine list featuring 650 selections that include many limited production and library wines.

The following recipe was created by Dry Creek Kitchen's executive chef, Michael Voltaggio, who says that his interest in cooking began at an early age growing up in Maryland. His first experience in restaurants came when he bused tables for his then sous-chef older brother Bryan, who is also in the Charlie Palmer organization. Chef Voltaggio went on to apprentice at the Greenbrier Hotel in West Virginia, trained under celebrity chef Larry Forgione at An American Place in New York City and The James Beard tribute restaurant, The Coach House. From there he moved to Florida to be sous-chef at the prestigious Ritz Carlton Hotel in Naples. Later he was promoted to chef de cuisine of the Dining Room restaurant and won the Ritz' Rising Chef award in 2004.

In talking about his recent move to California, he says that the local farmers and purveyors who come through his door on a daily basis are helping to make his adjustment an easy one. Chef Voltaggio states, "The earth-to-the-table relationship in Sonoma County is amazing to work with. I don't miss the Fed Ex charges to get great product either!"

Hotel Healdsburg
25 Matheson Street
Healdsburg, CA 95448
800-889-7188
www.hotelhealdsburg.com

Dry Creek Kitchen
317 Healdsburg Avenue
Healdsburg, CA 95448
707-431-0330
www.charliepalmer.com

Recipe from the Dry Creek Kitchen

by Executive Chef Michael Voltaggio

Fuyu Persimmon Carpaccio, Dry Creek Fig Dressing, Love Farm's Organic Greens & Spiced Brioche Croutons

Serves 4 as an appetizer

    4 Fuyu persimmons
    ¼ pound mixed fresh greens: sorrel, arugula, baby lettuces

Spiced Brioche Croutons
    ¼ cup clarified butter, warm
    ½ teaspoon each cinnamon, sugar, ground coriander seed, salt
    1 cup diced brioche (a rich French bread)

Dry Creek Fig Dressing
    1 tablespoon minced shallots
    1 cup cider vinegar
    ¾ cup Xeres Sherry wine vinegar
    1 cup water
    1 cup white wine
    1½ cups dried figs, small stems removed
    1 tablespoon Dijon mustard
    ½ cup extra-virgin olive oil

A note on buying persimmons: Persimmons must be absolutely ripe to be edible. There is no worse a culinary experience than sinking your teeth into an unripe persimmon, whose astringency rages a virtual war inside the mouth. The transformation the fruit makes from evil to sublime is a miraculous one. The fruit should be soft to the touch and only develops more of its honey-like sweetness with further ripening.

To prepare the croutons, preheat your oven to 300 degrees. Mix together the clarified butter and spices. Toss the diced brioche in the spiced butter until they are evenly coated and then lay them out flat on a cookie sheet.

Toast until golden brown in the oven, approximately 7 minutes. Remove the croutons from the oven when they have just lightly colored, as they will continue to color a bit from the butter. Let cool at room temperature.

To prepare the dressing, sweat the shallots with a bit of the olive oil with a pinch of salt in a sauce pot, large enough to accommodate all of the ingredients. Add the vinegars, water, and wine. Bring to a simmer and add the figs. Cook just until the mixture comes back to a simmer and then remove from the fire. Cover with plastic film and let stand until the ingredients have reached room temperature and the figs have been plumped by the cooking liquid.

Add the reconstituted figs to a blender along with any residual liquid left in the pot. Also add the mustard. Puree the mixture until smooth Then add the olive oil in a slow drizzle.

To assemble the dish, slice the persimmons into rounds about 1/8 of an inch thick. Lay them out onto plates in an overlapping pattern to form a circle. Season with salt and freshly ground pepper. Drizzle some of the fig vinaigrette abstractly over the persimmons.

Dress the greens with just enough of the fig vinaigrette to coat, and then mound small salads into the middles of each of the plates.

Scatter the croutons over the persimmons and serve.

Nutrition pyramid servings: Croutons, .75 grain, 90 pleasure food calories. Dressing, 1.5 fruit. Persimmons and greens, .75 fruit

Chef's wine suggestion: Dry Creek Vineyard Reserve Sauvignon Blanc

This beautiful and absolutely delicious dish is the perfect way to impress your friends or to delight your family. It is surprisingly easy to make, and if you prepare the full dressing recipe you will have lots left over for other salads. My eighteen-year-old son fell in love with the croutons and has been making them for his friends ever since. "Clarified butter," also known as "drawn butter," refers to unsalted butter that has been slowly melted, which evaporates most of the water and separates the milk solids. Skim any foam off the top, and pour the clear butter off the milky residue to use for the croutons.

Heading south from Healdsburg we come to the county's largest city, Santa Rosa. This city of 147,000 was ranked by *Forbes* magazine as number two in its list of the top ten most dynamic economic regions in the nation in 2002. In addition to the many wineries in the area, there are attractions such as the Luther Burbank Home and Gardens and historic Railroad Square. Vintner's Inn is located in Santa Rosa but feels far away from this bustling city. Next to their ninety-two-acre vineyard, the owners of Ferrari-Carano vineyards and winery, Don and Rhonda Carano, have sought to create a European-style hostelry with an atmosphere of luxury and serenity.

Adjacent to the inn is the area's most acclaimed restaurant, John Ash & Co. The restaurant got its start in the 1980s, during the time when California chefs like Alice Waters in Berkeley and John Ash in Sonoma County were refining wine country cuisine by rejecting traditional heavy sauces and developing a culinary approach that emphasizes seasonal, locally grown ingredients with light sauces that enhance the foods' natural flavors.

While John Ash has turned his attention now to writing and educating, his culinary philosophy continues at the restaurant under the direction of Executive Chef Jeffrey Madura, who added his own personal style to the menu. Chef Madura began his career at Mudd's Restaurant in San Ramon, California, which has its own two-acre organic garden. This led him to enroll at the California Culinary Academy and to work under John Ash. From there he went to work at the Royal Park Hotel in Tokyo and at Marriott Hotels in both London and Amsterdam. Coming back home he took the reins at his mentor's former restaurant, John Ash & Co., where on a warm summer's night you can enjoy his innovative and highly praised menu out on the terrace overlooking the vineyards.

Vintner's Inn
4350 Barnes Road
Santa Rosa, CA 95405
800-421-2584
www.vintnersinn.com

John Ash & Co.
4330 Barnes Road
Santa Rosa, CA 95403
707-527-7687
www.johnashrestaurant.com

Recipes from John Ash & Co.

by Executive Chef Jeffrey Madura

Roasted Pork Loin Stuffed with Caramelized Fennel, Red Onion, and Watercress—Served with a Watercress Salad with an Orange and Pink Peppercorn Vinaigrette

Serves 12

Roasted Pork Loin

6 6-ounce pork tenderloins, trimmed and cleaned, hollowed out with a sharpening steel for stuffing. (can be cut in half to make 12 3-ounce servings)

1 medium fennel bulb, cored and cut into 1-inch dice

1 medium red onion cut into ¼-inch dice

2 bunches watercress leaves, washed, picked and cut in julienne strips

3 tablespoons clarified butter or olive oil

Ground pepper to taste

Kosher salt to taste

¼ cup olive oil

After cleaning and trimming pork tenderloins, place a sharpening steel into the center of each pork tenderloin to create a pocket for stuffing.

In a large sauté pan, heat clarified butter until hot. Add diced fennel and red onion and coat well with butter. Caramelize the onion mixture on high flame for 8 to 12 minutes.

Once caramelized, cool mixture down, add watercress and season with salt and pepper. Mix well. Then stuff ¼ cup of this mixture into each pork tenderloin cavity.

Once all are stuffed, marinate in olive oil, and salt and pepper until ready to cook.

Heat sauté pan with olive oil or heat grill and cook pork tenderloins until medium—about 8 to 10 minutes. Once cooked, let stand to retain juices and heat.

While the tenderloins sit, make the salad and dressing.

Orange and Pink Peppercorn Vinaigrette

6 ounces unsweetened frozen orange juice concentrate
1/3 cup low-sodium soy sauce
¼ cup rice wine vinegar
1 tablespoon peeled and minced fresh ginger
1½ teaspoons dark sesame oil
½ cup scallions, white and pale green parts
¼ cup chopped fresh Italian flat leaf parsley
1 cup olive or peanut oil
¼ cup dry toasted pink peppercorns

In a food processor or blender, combine all ingredients except the oil and pink peppercorns. Process until smooth. Transfer to a bowl.

Stir in the oil and peppercorns being careful not to emulsify, otherwise the dressing will be too thick.

Store any unused dressing covered and refrigerated for up to two weeks.

Watercress Salad
Serves 12

2 medium fennel bulbs, thinly sliced vertically in 1/6-inch strips
2 medium red onions, thinly sliced in rings and shocked in cold water for 10 minutes
2 bunches watercress, stemmed and cleaned
2 blood or navel oranges peeled and sliced into thin rounds ¼ inch thick

Kosher salt and black pepper to taste

Arrange salad by mixing shaved fennel, red onion, and watercress in stainless steel bowl. Add kosher salt and ground black pepper to taste, and arrange attractively on large platters. Add orange rounds to each bunch to give height.

Cut tenderloins into 12 pieces and arrange on individual platters next to salad mixture. Drizzle with orange and pink peppercorn vinaigrette, and garnish with fennel frond.

Nutrition pyramid servings: Pork loin = 3 meat, .5 vegetable, 1 oil; watercress salad lightly tossed with dressing = 1 vegetable, 1.5 oil

Chef's wine suggestion: Bonny Doon Cigare Blanc (Rhone blend)

Pork is a wonderfully lean meat, and this recipe makes a delicious pork tenderloin that is fairly easy to prepare. Get a tenderloin that is thick enough for stuffing, and be careful not to overcook it as I did the first time. Cook it until an instant-read thermometer registers 135 to 140 degrees. As the tenderloin rests, the internal temperature will come up to 145 to 150 degrees and will be within the temperature range for safe eating. This recipe can be cut in half to yield six servings. Plans B and C will have one whole pork loin.

Watermelon and Red Onion Salad

1 tablespoon chopped shallots

1/3 cup raspberry vinegar

1/3 cup fresh or frozen raspberries, puréed and strained

2 teaspoons honey or to taste

1/3 cup olive oil

Kosher salt and freshly ground black pepper

2 medium red onions, thinly sliced

2 bunches watercress, stems removed

8 cups watermelon cut into 1-inch cubes. Use both red and yellow watermelon if available.

Garnish: julienned mint leaves

In a medium bowl, whisk together the shallots, vinegar, raspberry purée, honey, and oil. Season to taste with salt and pepper.

Separate the onions into rings. Pour the vinaigrette over the onions and marinate in the refrigerator for at least 15 minutes.

To serve, arrange a bed of watercress on each chilled plate. Top with the cubed watermelon and drape the onion rings on top. Drizzle with the vinaigrette and garnish with the mint leaves if desired.

Nutrition pyramid servings: 1 vegetable, 1 fruit, 2 oil

Chef's wine suggestion: Kosta-Brown Pinot Noir Rosé

While it is possible to get watermelon these days in other seasons, this is definitely a salad for a warm summer day when the watermelons are ripe, fresh, and sweet. It is hard to imagine beforehand just what a wonderful combination this light salad of watermelon, red onion, raspberry, and mint makes.

While John Ash is busy traveling around the country teaching and writing, he still calls Sonoma County home.

Recipes by Chef John Ash

Corn Soup with Crab

Serves 4

2 tablespoons butter
1½ cups chopped onion (1 medium)
1 cup chopped carrots
¼ cup chopped celery
2 teaspoons chopped garlic
3½ cups or so corn kernels (cut from 6 medium ears)
1 whole star anise or bay leaf
5 cups de-fatted chicken stock
Salt and freshly ground pepper
½ pound fresh Dungeness or lump crabmeat, picked over
2 tablespoons finely chopped chives

In a deep saucepan or soup pot, heat the butter over moderate heat. Add the onion, carrots, celery, and garlic and cook till soft but not brown, about 5 minutes, stirring occasionally. Add the corn, star anise, and saffron and continue to cook and stir for another 5 minutes.

Add the stock and bring to a boil. Reduce heat to a simmer and cook for 10 minutes. Discard the star anise or bay leaf and puree in a blender being careful to do so at a lower speed and with blender jar only half filled. (Hot liquids expand dramatically, so be careful.) You'll need to do this in batches.

Strain the soup through a medium-mesh strainer by pushing down on the solids and return to the pan. Season with salt and pepper and reheat. Ladle into warm soup bowls, top with the crab and chives, and serve.

Recipe © 2004 John Ash

Nutrition pyramid servings: 1.5 grain, 1 vegetable, 1 meat, 45 pleasure food calories

Chef's wine suggestions: "I'd choose one of the aromatic varietals (Riesling, Gewurztraminer, Viognier, Muscat, or Sauvignon Blanc) for both the soup and the salad and preferably one that had just a touch of residual sugar in it. Also choose one with no oak aging."

John Ash says, "This healthy recipe calls for crab but you could use whatever sweet shellfish is available to you, such as lobster or shrimp. If you wanted to go 'whole hog' you could, of course, garnish with a squiggle of crème fraiche, caviar, etcetera!"

While best when the summer corn is ripe, this delicious soup is also wonderful on a cold winter evening using frozen corn. It takes a bit of time to prepare but is well worth it.

Warm Red Cabbage Salad with Pancetta and California Goat Cheese

Serves 6

1/3 pound good-quality pancetta, cut into ¼-inch dice

2 teaspoons roasted garlic

2 tablespoons wild honey or to taste

¼ cup champagne vinegar

½ cup olive oil

Salt and fresh ground black pepper to taste

1 pound red cabbage, cored and finely shredded

4–6 ounces California soft ripening or aged goat cheese, cut in attractive shapes

Garnish: Sunflower or daikon sprouts if desired

Add the pancetta to a sauté pan along with ¾ cup water and cook over moderate heat until water evaporates and pancetta browns—about 8 minutes. Be sure to stir to brown evenly. Remove and set aside. In the same sauté pan, add the garlic, honey, and vinegar together and then slowly whisk in the olive oil. Season to your taste with salt and pepper.

Heat the sauté pan over moderate-high heat. Add the cabbage and toss quickly for a minute or 2 just to warm through. Stir in the pancetta. Place on warm plates. Arrange the goat cheese on top, along with sprouts, and serve immediately.

JOHN ASH © 1989 REV. 1/05

Nutrition pyramid servings: 1 vegetable, 3.5 oil, 1 dairy

Chef's wine suggestion: See above under Corn Soup with Crab recipe

John Ash says, "For the goat cheese I especially like the Bucheret, Camellia or Crottin from Redwood Hill Farms (www.redwoodhillfarms. com) or the Humboldt Fog or Bermuda Triangle from Cypress Grove (www. cypressgrovechevre.com)."

I really love this salad. It is so rich and filled with a variety of taste sensations. With some good bread it can be a whole meal. Pancetta is an Italian bacon that is cured with salt and spices but not smoked. It comes in a sausage-like roll.

Located just off the square in the town of Sonoma is Café La Haye, a restaurant loved by locals and tourists alike, which serves well-prepared, wholesome food from its tiny open kitchen. It is co-owned by John McReynolds and Saul Gropman. *Zagat Guides* describes Café La Haye as being like "a fine vintage" that "just keeps getting better and better." Chef

McReynolds was trained at the California Culinary Academy in San Francisco and went on to work in a number of unique settings. These included a year on a private yacht sailing in the Mediterranean, a dude ranch in Colorado, and establishing the food service at Skywalker Ranch, the Lucas Film complex in Marin County. McReynolds describes the process of creating menus and cooking as "intensely gratifying and fun."

> Café La Haye
> 140 E. Napa Street
> Sonoma, CA 95476
> (707) 935-5994
> www.cafelahaye.com

Recipes from the Café La Haye

by Chef John McReynolds

Mache and Spring Vegetable Salad with Goat Cheese and Tapenade Toast

Serves 4

> ½ pound mache
> ¼ pound asparagus
> 1 fennel bulb
> ¼ pound baby carrots
> 1 red pepper
> 6 ounces goat cheese
> 4 slices country sourdough bread
> 4 ounces tapenade
> Citrus vinaigrette

Tapenade

> ¼ cup pitted black olives
> 2 tablespoons capers
> 2 cloves garlic minced
> 1 teaspoon grated orange zest
> 2 anchovy filets finely chopped

½ teaspoon pepper

½ cup green olive oil (green olive oil is extra-virgin oil that is pressed before the olives are ripe and is more pungent and peppery—any extra-virgin olive oil can be used)

Place all ingredients in food processor and pulse 3 times.

Vinaigrette

1 tablespoon lemon juice

2 tablespoons orange juice

2 tablespoons champagne vinegar

2 shallots finely chopped

2 tablespoons green olive oil

4 tablespoons canola oil

Lemon and orange zest

Salt and pepper

Wash and dry mache. Peel and blanch asparagus. Peel and blanch carrots. Roast and peel pepper. Shave fennel. Slice bread, brush with olive oil, and grill on both sides. Spread tapenade on bread. Toss vegetables with vinaigrette and reserve. Toss mache with vinaigrette and divide evenly between 4 plates. Arrange vegetables on top of mache. Crumble goat cheese over each salad. Serve with tapenade toasts.

Nutrition pyramid servings: Salad = 2 vegetable, 1 oil, 1 dairy;

Bread = 1 grain; 1 tablespoon tapenade = 2 oil; 2 teaspoons vinaigrette = 1 oil

Chef's wine suggestion: "Acidic foods are usually a good match with Sauvignon Blanc. The earth flavors of this salad need to be matched with a wine with tart but balanced acidity. Ingredients that go well with Sauvignon Blanc are olives, goat cheese, red pepper, herbs, pepper, fish, shellfish, some poultry, as well as Mediterranean and Middle Eastern foods."

Mache, also called Lamb's Lettuce, is becoming easier to find in grocery stores. Pronounced "mosh," mache is a delicate succulent green with graceful, velvety leaves. This is a delightful salad that easily makes for a full meal. While the preparation takes a while, the bonus is that all the ingredients can be used for future treats. The vegetables go well in an omelet the next day, and the vinaigrette can be used for other salads. Best of all is the tapenade, which makes a great spread for bread and crackers.

Chilled Cucumber Soup with Red Pepper Coulis

Serves 6

Chilled Cucumber Soup

3 pounds cucumber—peeled and seeded

Juice of 3 lemons

½ quart cold vegetable stock

Kosher salt and white pepper to taste

½ cup nonfat yogurt (optional)

Puree all ingredients together with blender or handheld blender. Strain through a coarse strainer. Allow to cool several hours in refrigerator. Taste for seasoning before serving in cold bowls.

Red Pepper Coulis

1 red sweet pepper, fire-roasted, peeled and seeded

Juice 1 lemon

1 tablespoon capers

3 tablespoons olive oil

Salt and pepper to taste

Puree all ingredients in food processor until very smooth. Drizzle on top of soup. Garnish with chives and chive oil.

Nutrition pyramid servings: 1 vegetable, 1.5 oil

Chef's wine suggestion: Viognier

This soup is perfect for a warm evening. The contrast between the cucumber soup and the red pepper coulis is an agreeable surprise. It is a perfect recipe to make ahead of time. You can grill the red pepper yourself, or, if you're short on time, you can buy jars of red peppers already prepared.

Seared Wild Salmon with Cherry Tomato Vinaigrette

Serves 8–16

8 6-ounce pieces of salmon filet

1 pound cherry tomatoes, rinsed, dried, and halved

½ red onion finely chopped

2 ounces Champagne vinegar

Juice 1 lemon

2 ounces canola oil

2 ounces extra-virgin olive oil

1 ounce of mixed finely chopped herbs (parsley, chervil, chives, tarragon)

Salt and pepper

Liberally season salmon pieces with salt and pepper. In a bowl, mix tomatoes, onions, salt, pepper, and vinegar. Allow to macerate (soak) for 30 minutes. Add oil and herbs.

Preheat oven to 400 degrees.

Heat cast iron skillet to very hot. Pour small amount of oil in pan and sear 2 pieces of salmon at a time on both sides. Place salmon on baking pan, and put in preheated oven for 5 minutes.

Place salmon on plate and top with vinaigrette.

Serve with roasted corn; cut off the cob.

Nutrition pyramid servings: Full portion: 6 meat, 1 vegetable, 3 oil; half portion: 3 meat, .5 vegetable, 1.5 oil

Chef's wine suggestion: "I like Pinot Noir with salmon. A second choice would be a rosé."

This is a light and easy way to serve salmon. With the addition of the corn, you have a complete meal.

Napa County

www.napavalley.com
www.winecountry.com

Recognized as one of the finest viticulture regions in the world, Napa Valley is home to more than 200 wineries. Only thirty miles long and five miles wide, it is the least populated county in the Bay Area. At the north end of the county is Calistoga, known for its mud baths and spas, and at the southern end, the town of Napa. Other communities include Saint Helena, Rutherford, Oakville, and Yountville. While grapes have been grown commercially here since the 1840s, it was not until the 1960s and 1970s that the county began to attain its present acclaim.

The economy of Napa County is now based on wine and tourism. Many celebrities have also been drawn to the wine-country lifestyle delights of Napa. Property owners in the Valley include Francis Ford Coppola, Robin Williams, Robert Redford, and Joe Montana.

The town of Napa is undergoing a renaissance, triggered by a multimillion dollar flood-control project along the Napa River and the development of COPIA: The American Center for Wine, Food & the Arts. In 1988, legendary vintner Robert Mondavi, with his wife, Margit Biever Mondavi, and other leaders in the wine community, began to explore the idea of creating a small institution to celebrate achievements in the culinary and winemaking arts. The concept evolved into a major nonprofit cultural institution devoted to exploring food, wine, and the arts.

In 1996, Mondavi purchased twelve acres of land on the Napa River and was instrumental in raising the $55 million needed to complete the building of COPIA, named for the goddess of abundance. Its doors were opened to the public on November 18, 2001.

There is something for everyone to enjoy at COPIA—from touring the organic Edible Gardens and exploring exhibitions to participating in wine and food programs, tastings, festivals, and fun children's programs. Special seasonal events held throughout the year include "Chocolate Passion" in February and summer's "Berry Bonanza." The Wine Spectator Tasting Table presents daily wine tastings, and every Friday there's a Taste of COPIA lunch featuring seasonal dishes and wine pairings. For dining at COPIA, you have two settings to choose from: Julia's Kitchen for fine cuisine and the American Market Café for casual fare.

Julia's Kitchen is named after Julia Child, who was an honorary trustee and invaluable advisor to COPIA's development. She also donated her copper cookware collection from her home in Cambridge, Massachusetts, which is on display in COPIA's core exhibition, Forks in the Road.

The following recipes were created by COPIA Culinary Instructor Jill Silverman Hough, who says that she spent her first career as an advertising copywriter, thinking up clever headlines for everything from diapers to credit cards. For a second career, she owned a café that made, among other things, "the world's best chocolate chip cookies." Her third career, as a Napa-based freelance food writer, recipe developer, and instructor at COPIA perfectly combines her first two careers.

Jill's column, "Quick Cuisine," appears in *ANG* newspapers semi-monthly. She also writes for magazines such as *Bon Appetit* and is working on a cookbook. "My style is simple yet special," says Jill. "Cooking doesn't have to be complicated to be indulgent."

COPIA: The American Center for Wine, Food & the Arts
500 First Street
Napa, CA 94559
www.copia.org
707-259-1600

Recipes from COPIA: The American Center for Wine, Food & the Arts

by Jill Silverman Hough

Polenta and Grilled Vegetable Napoleons with Ricotta Salata, Grilled Corn and Basil Vinaigrette

Serves 6

    Vegetable oil
    1½ quarts water
    3 tablespoons kosher salt, plus more for seasoning
    3 tablespoons extra virgin olive oil, plus more for brushing
    12 ounces polenta

¾ cup freshly grated Parmigiano-Reggiano cheese

1 globe eggplant, cut into ¼-inch slices

5 sweet peppers, cut lengthwise into thirds, ribs and seeds removed

2 red onions, cut into ¼-inch slices

Black pepper

1 ear corn, shucked

3 tomatoes, cut into ¼-inch slices

¾ pound part-skim ricotta salata, crumbled

Basil vinaigrette (see recipe below)

Basil leaves for garnish

Polenta

Lightly coat two 9" x 13" baking pans with vegetable oil. In a large pot, bring the water to a boil. Add the salt and olive oil. Add the polenta in a slow stream, stirring constantly. Lower the temperature. Cook the polenta for 15 to 20 minutes, stirring occasionally with a wooden spoon. Remove from the heat and stir in the Parmigiano-Reggiano cheese. Spread the polenta onto the prepared baking sheets and allow to cool. Refrigerate overnight or until firm.

Grilled Polenta and Vegetables

Prepare a grill to medium hot. Cut each pan of polenta into 9 rectangles, for a total of 18 pieces. Brush both sides of each piece of polenta with a generous amount of olive oil. Brush both sides of the eggplant slices, peppers, and onions with olive oil. Brush corn with olive oil. Generously season all vegetables with salt and pepper.

Grill polenta until lightly charred on both sides, 6 to 8 minutes per side. (Be very careful turning the polenta over—use a metal spatula and make sure it releases before you flip it—if it sticks, it's most likely not charred enough.) Grill eggplant, peppers, and onions until softened and lightly charred on both sides, 3 to 6 minutes per side. (It's tricky turning the onion slices over—it's okay if a few of them fall through the grates.) Grill corn until it is lightly charred on all sides, 10 to 12 minutes.

To assemble the Napoleons: When the corn is cool enough to handle, cut off the kernels. Place a piece of grilled polenta in the center of 6 plates. Top each piece of polenta with a slice of tomato, a slice of eggplant, a piece of pepper, and a slice of onion. Repeat all layers—polenta, tomato, eggplant, pepper, and onion. Finish with a final piece of polenta. Cut the remaining peppers into thin slices. Top each Napoleon with a small tangle of sliced peppers. Sprinkle corn and the ricotta salata over the top of each Napoleon. Drizzle each with about 2 tablespoons of basil vinaigrette, garnish with a basil leaf, and serve.

Basil Vinaigrette
1 cup packed basil leaves
½ cup white wine vinegar
1 tablespoon sugar
1 teaspoon kosher salt, or more to taste
¼ teaspoon black pepper, or more to taste
1 cup extra-virgin olive oil

In a food processor, puree basil, white wine vinegar, sugar, salt and pepper. With the motor running, slowly drizzle in olive oil. Taste and adjust seasonings.

© Copia: The American Center for Wine, Food & the Arts (2005). Recipe developed by Jill Hough, COPIA culinary instructor.

Nutrition pyramid servings: Polenta: 1 grain, 1 vegetable, .5 oil, .5 dairy; basil vinaigrette: 1 tablespoon = 2.5 oil

Chef's wine suggestion: La Rocca Vineyards White Zinfandel or Bonny Doon Ca'del Solo Big House Red.

You are in for an extraordinary indulgence with these vegetable Napoleons. They are both beautiful to look at and delightful to taste. You can save some time by purchasing already prepared polenta or roasted red peppers. Make sure to slice the eggplant thinly. If you cannot find ricotta salata cheese, use a mild feta or goat cheese. To minimize oil, spray polenta and veggies with olive oil instead of brushing with olive oil.

Great Garden-Inspired Grilled Chicken

Serves 12 (3–4 ounces each)
1 cup balsamic vinegar
3/4 cup extra-virgin olive oil
1 tablespoon honey

1½ teaspoons salt, or more to taste

1 teaspoon chopped fresh or dried lavender

1 teaspoon chopped fresh rosemary

1¼ teaspoon freshly ground pepper, or more to taste

6 6- to 8-ounce boneless skinless chicken breast halves, washed, trimmed, and dried

Whisk together the balsamic vinegar, olive oil, honey, salt, lavender, rosemary, and pepper. Place the chicken in a large, resealable bag and add vinegar mixture. Let stand at least 2 hours, or as long as overnight.

Prepare a grill to medium-high heat. Drain the chicken and discard marinade. Place the chicken directly onto the grate. Cook for 2 to 3 minutes per side or until just opaque throughout. Cut breasts in half and serve.

Serving suggestions

- Place chicken breasts on a bed of arugula with a drizzle of good-quality balsamic vinegar and a sprinkle of lavender.
- Slice chicken and toss with mixed greens, crumbled goat cheese and diced nectarines.
- Serve chicken on a bed of Israeli couscous and top with chopped sun-dried tomatoes and a sprig of rosemary.

© Copia: The American Center for Wine, Food & the Arts (2005). Recipe developed by Jill Hough, COPIA culinary instructor.

Nutrition pyramid servings: 3–4 meat, 1 oil

This is an easy and tasty way to prepare chicken breasts that can go equally well in a salad or as part of a warm dinner. Be sure to make extra for future meals.

COPIA Garden Berry Sorbet

Serves 16

2½ pounds ripe berries—all one kind or a mixture—stems removed

2 cups simple syrup, or to taste (see recipe below)

3 tablespoons freshly squeezed lemon or lime juice, or to taste.

Pinch of salt

If using blueberries, cook them over medium-high heat in a large non-reactive pot with a bit of water until they are very soft. Allow berries to cool before continuing.

With an immersion blender or in a food processor, thoroughly puree the berries. Strain the puree through a medium-mesh sieve. Stir in the simple syrup, juice, and salt. Taste the sorbet and add more syrup, juice, or salt if necessary. Freeze according to ice-cream-maker manufacturer's directions.

Simple syrup
4 cups sugar
4 cups water

Combine sugar and water in a medium saucepan and heat just to the boil. Remove from heat and let cool. Simple syrup can be infused with flavor by steeping it with herbs or spices.

© Copia: The American Center for Wine, Food & the Arts (2005). Recipe developed by Jill Hough, COPIA culinary instructor.

Nutrition pyramid servings: .5 fruit, 100 pleasure food calories

What a wonderful way to turn fresh fruit into a special dessert that everyone in the family will enjoy. The directions are easy to follow. Take out your ice-cream maker and enjoy.

ZuZu is a small and lively tapas restaurant located in Napa's historic Old Town district and beloved by loyal locals. Chef Angela Tamura and proprietor Mick Salyer describe their philosophy as simply being, "Great food, great friends, and great fun." The warm, cozy atmosphere and Latin music in the background help create an environment where food, wine, art, and friends are all celebrated.

ZuZu serves a variety of small flavorful plates that are meant to be shared around the table. Menu items change every month with an eye to always keeping within the season. Using only seasonal, organic ingredients, there is something for every palate from Moroccan Glazed Lamb Chops to Rainbow Chard with Golden Raisins and Pine Nuts to Saffron Scented Spanish Paella. Jordan MacKay of *Wine & Spirits* says, "The Gods were smiling on me as they led me to ZuZu."

Chef Tamura is a graduate of the New England Culinary Institute in Vermont and has been cooking her entire life in one form or another. She has worked in many fine restaurants including Rialto in Cambridge, Massachusetts, the Ritz-Carlton on Amelia Island, and Bistro Don Giovanni in Napa.

ZuZu Restaurant
829 Main Street, Napa, CA 94559
707-224-8555
www.zuzunapa.com

Recipes from the ZuZu Restaurant
by Chef Angela Tamura

Pan-Seared Halibut with Red Pepper Romesco

Serves 8

> 8 3-ounce portions halibut
> ½ head cauliflower
> 1 cup romesco sauce
> Canola oil for searing
> ½ bunch parsley, chopped
> 1 lemon
> 1 tablespoon extra-virgin olive oil
> Salt and pepper

Romesco Sauce

Serves 8

> 4 red peppers, roasted, peeled, and seeded
> 1 pasilla pepper, reconstituted in hot water and pureed
> 2 roasted tomatoes, peeled
> ¼ cup roasted garlic cloves
> ¼ cup hazelnuts
> ¼ cup day-old bread, toasted
> ¼ cup sherry vinegar
> ¼ cup extra-virgin olive oil
> Salt and pepper

Combine the ingredients in the bowl of a food processor and taste for seasoning. Use any leftovers as a salad dressing, sandwich spread, or sauce.

Break the cauliflower into bite-sized florets and blanch in boiling, salted water for 4 minutes. Remove the florets to a small baking sheet and roast in a 400 degree oven for five minutes or until slightly crispy.

Meanwhile, heat the canola oil in a large frying pan until almost smoking. Season the fish and place into pan. Do not move the fish once you have placed it in the oil, but leave it until you can see a nice crust start to form. Flip the fish once, and then cook it briefly in the oven until just cooked—roughly 5 minutes. Be careful not to overcook the halibut as it will dry out.

On each of 5 plates, spoon a little of the romesco sauce. Toss the cauliflower with the juice of half the lemon and the olive oil and mound on top of the sauce. Finally place the halibut portions on top; squeeze with lemon and garnish with parsley.

Nutrition pyramid servings: Halibut: 3 meat, .5 vegetable, .5 oil. Sauce: 1 vegetable, 2 oil

This makes a delectable complete dinner. If halibut is not in season, try another white fish such as cod. The pasilla pepper can be found in the Latin food section.

Golden Beet Salad with Blood Oranges and Banyuls Vinaigrette

Serves 4

2 medium golden beets
1 cup orange juice
½ cup white wine
½ each cinnamon stick
2 pieces star anise
2 blood oranges
1 cup mache
½ cup walnuts, toasted
Salt and pepper to taste
¼ bunch parsley, chopped
12 endive spears

Banyuls Vinaigrette
½ tablespoon Banyuls vinegar
1 teaspoon Champagne vinegar
1½ tablespoons canola oil
2 tablespoons walnut oil

Preheat oven to 400 degrees. In a small oven-safe dish, place the beets, orange juice, wine, cinnamon, and star anise and roast for approximately 1 hour or until the beets are tender. Remove them from the oven and allow to cool to room temperature.

While the beets are cooling, peel the oranges with a knife by cutting off the two ends and cutting down between the flesh and the skin; be careful to remove all of the pith as you cut. Section the oranges with your knife by cutting down either side of the segment in a "V." In a small bowl mix together the ingredients for the dressing and set aside.

Peel the beets using a towel to rub off the skin, and cut into bite-sized squares.

In a small bowl toss together the beets, blood orange segments, mache, walnuts, parsley, and vinaigrette and taste for salt and pepper. Place 3 spears of endive on each of 4 plates and then gently spoon the salad on top.

Chef Tamura describes this as "a wonderfully earthy salad which uses a sweet wine vinegar from France." She adds, "Although it adds a few more calories, at the restaurant we cannot resist candying the walnuts. First, simmer together the juice of the 2 blood oranges with 2 tablespoons of granulated sugar and reduce by half, then add the walnuts to it and cook for several minutes. Remove the nuts to a bowl and toss with 1 teaspoon of sugar and a dash of cinnamon. Bake for 10 minutes at 375 degrees."

Nutrition pyramid servings: Golden beet salad: 2 vegetable, 1 nut, .5 fruit; vinaigrette: 2.5 oil. If candying walnuts add 27 pleasure food calories.

You will greatly enjoy this sweet and nutritious beet salad. It easily can be a main course. If you are not able to find the Banyuls vinegar, use another ½ tablespoon of Champagne vinegar.

Alameda County

www.acgov.com
www.insideBayArea.com

Driving south from Napa on Highway 29 we leave the countryside behind and come to the populous San Francisco Bay area. South of Berkeley and Oakland and east of San Francisco lie two wine producing areas that date back to the earliest days of California history—southern Alameda County and northern Santa Clara County. Wineries such as Concannon, Wente, and Mirassou date back more than a century. Livermore Valley, off Interstate 580 in southern Alameda County, has managed to evade suburban invasion through agricultural preserves that have been established to protect vineyards. The Livermore Valley was settled by an English sailor, Robert Livermore, who picked up two Mexican land grants in 1830 and began grape growing shortly thereafter.

After learning about winemaking from Charles Krug, Charles Heinrich Wente, a first-generation immigrant from Germany, founded his own winery in 1883, in the Livermore Valley, and, in 1918, his sons Ernest and Herman joined the business. Today Wente Vineyards is managed by the fourth generation of the Wente family and includes over 2,000 acres of vineyards. The beautiful grounds of the Wente Vineyards Restaurant and Visitors Center include a golf course, lawns, and an herb garden from which seasonings are picked for the nearby restaurant. In addition to the tasting room, there is a small museum and 650 feet of aging caves which visitors can explore. The restaurant opens onto the lush vineyards and gardens through French doors. The Wente philosophy for menu planning and preparation is one of "honesty, simplicity, and integrity." It features "American dishes, influenced by Italian, French, and California cuisine" —with wine in mind.

Wente Vineyards Restaurant & Visitors Center
5050 Arroyo Road
Livermore, CA 94550
(925) 456-2450
www.wentevineyards.com

Recipes from the Wente Vineyards Restaurant
by Chef Elisabeth Schwarz

Wood-Fired Heirloom Tomato Soup with Little Croutons

4 servings

> 5–6 large Heirloom tomatoes
> 1 medium-size red onion
> 2 cloves garlic
> ½ bunch basil leaves
> 4 teaspoon olive oil
> Salt and pepper
> Balsamic vinegar
> 4 slices bread, cubed and toasted

Preheat charcoal grill. Core tomatoes and cut in half horizontally. Shake out seeds. Peel and thickly slice red onion.

Brush tomatoes and red onion with oil. Season with salt and pepper to taste. Place cut side down onto grill.

Meanwhile, slice garlic cloves and sauté with 1 teaspoon olive oil over medium heat.

Grill the tomatoes and the red onion until they become lightly charred. Place tomatoes, onion, and garlic into a large pot. Rough chop basil leaves and add. Puree this combination with a handheld blender until smooth. Season with salt and pepper to taste.

If desired, a splash of balsamic vinegar can be added for further seasoning. Pass the soup through a strainer.

This soup can be served hot or chilled. Serve with the croutons.

Nutrition pyramid servings: 1 grain, 2.5 vegetable, 1 oil

Chef's wine suggestion: Zinfandel.

This is tomato soup that will spoil your enjoyment of the canned variety forever. While it certainly is best with Heirloom tomatoes on a grill, we couldn't wait for summer and made a great version in January using organic tomatoes and the broiler. With a slice of sourdough bread and a green salad, it makes an easy-to-prepare meal any season of the year. To reduce oil, spray on olive oil instead of brushing vegetables, and sauté in a skillet coated with oil spray.

Steamed Clams with Garlic, Chiles, Sauvignon Blanc, Spinach, Oregano, Parsley and Grilled Country Bread

Serves 4

> 40–50 littleneck clams
> 2 teaspoons garlic, finely chopped
> 2 serrano chiles, seeded, and finely sliced
> 2 jalapeno chiles, seeded, and finely sliced
> 1 cup Wente Vineyards Sauvignon Blanc
> 4 handsful baby spinach, washed
> 1 bunch oregano, finely chopped
> 1 bunch parsley, finely chopped
> 4 teaspoons olive oil
> 2 teaspoons butter (optional)
> Salt and pepper to taste

Heat skillet over medium-high heat and add oil. Into the hot pan add garlic and chiles. Stir to prevent garlic and chiles from sticking to the pan. Cool for 30 seconds. Add clams. Add white wine and cover pan. Steam clams this way for 3 to 4 minutes. Brush sliced bread with oil (optional), and sprinkle with salt and pepper. Grill or toast bread to desired doneness. Make sure that all clams have opened, and discard those which have not. Add spinach to pan, and briefly wilt into clams. Season with salt and pepper to taste. Add butter. Rub toasted bread with garlic while still warm. Serve alongside steamed clams.

Nutrition pyramid servings: 1 grain, 1 vegetable, 1 oil, 2 meat

Chef's wine suggestion: Sauvignon Blanc

This is another easy to prepare and unique dish from Chef Schwarz. The Sauvignon Blanc is a good balance with the hotness of the serrano and jalapeno chiles, which can be found fresh in the produce section. A light salad or steamed vegetable makes a good accompaniment.

Tuolumne County

www.tcchamber.com

www.columbiacalifornia.com

Before we head down the California coast, we're going take a side trip east to the California Gold Country. After traveling due east out of the Livermore Valley on Interstate 580 and then 205 to Stockton, take highways 120 and 108 up to Tuolumne County and the Sierra Nevada foothills. This area is renowned for its breathtaking vistas, recreational activities, and gold rush history. Within the area is Yosemite National Park, Stanislaus National Forest, Columbia and Railtown state historic parks, and a number of gold rush towns.

We're going to be stopping at Columbia State Historic Park and the town of Columbia, which has preserved its gold rush-era business district with shops, restaurants, and two hotels. Visitors can ride a 100-year-old stagecoach, pan for gold, and tour an active gold mine. Columbia's historic City Hotel has been beautifully restored and furnished with exquisite antiques. Special events at the hotel include a Victorian Christmas Feast, murder mystery weekends, winemaker dinners, and culinary arts classes. The restaurant at the hotel features gourmet dining with the freshest of California ingredients and a comprehensive wine list that includes numerous older vintages as well as a fascinating selection of Sierra foothill wines. Morgan's Restaurant at the City Hotel has been a recipient of the Wine Spectator Restaurant Award since 1986.

Executive Chef Jeff Zahniser refers with pride to his area of California as "the new wine country." He is a graduate of the Culinary Institute of America and a recipient of the Tabasco-McKelheny Award of Excellence. He was the co-host of "Cooking 'n Concert," a cooking and music television show in Santa Monica, California. After many years in his role as executive chef for several hotels and restaurants in Miami, New York, and Los Angeles, Zahniser decided that the time was right to make his dream a reality and make the big move to the Mother Lode. In addition to his work as a chef, he is culinary instructor for Columbia Community College's Hospitality Management Program.

City Hotel
Box 1870,
Columbia, CA 95310
(209) 532-1479
www.cityhotel.com

Recipes from Morgan's Restaurant at the City Hotel

by Chef Jeffrey Zahniser

Cornish Game Hen "Pot au Feu" with Winter Vegetables

Serves 1 (Multiply recipe by desired number of servings.)

1 Cornish game hen (4 ounces meat). Debone rib bones. Leg and wing bones remain, but remove the wing tips.

½ carrot, cut on the bias into ½-inch slices

1 potato, cubed

1 celery rib, peeled, and cut into 2-inch pieces

Salt

1 turnip, medium, peeled and quartered

1 leek, split in half, cleaned, cut in 2-inch pieces, use white part only

Black pepper, freshly ground

1 teaspoon Dijon mustard

1 tablespoon nonfat sour cream

½ teaspoon horseradish, freshly grated

Cornishons or gherkins, garnish (optional)

Wash the game hens, inside and out, with cold running water. Pat dry. Season and tie into a roll around the legs. Place in a large pot and add cold water or chicken stock to cover by about 3 inches. Bring to a boil over high heat. Reduce the heat to medium and simmer for 15 minutes, frequently skimming off any fat that rises to the top.

Add the carrots, celery, and leek. Season with salt. Simmer for 45 minutes. Add the turnips and simmer for 12 minutes. Taste and adjust the seasoning with salt and pepper.

Place the potatoes in a large saucepan and add cold water to cover by about 1 inch. Add a pinch of salt. Bring to a boil over high heat. Reduce the heat to medium and cook for 20 minutes or until tender when pierced with a fork. Drain well and keep warm.

In a small bowl, combine the sour cream and mustard. Whisk well. Fold in the horseradish. Transfer to a small serving bowl.

Remove the game hens from the broth and place on a plate to cool slightly. Keep the broth and vegetables warm.

Place the game hens in a soup tureen. Add the cooking broth.

Place the tureen on the table and ladle into individual shallow soup bowls. Pass the horseradish mixture to be used as a condiment. Garnish with cornishons or gherkins.

Nutrition pyramid servings: 4 meat, 5 vegetable

This is a delicious and fun dish that provides a full meal. If you do not want to debone the Cornish game hens, the recipe will still work fine. If you are unable to find fresh horseradish, use the same amount of bottled horseradish.

Crab Crowned Venison Medallions

Serves 6

12 3-ounce venison medallions

6 tablespoons canola oil

Pepper to taste

6 ounce crab meat

3 red bell peppers, fine dice

3 green bell peppers, fine dice

3 yellow bell peppers, fine dice

3 fennel bulbs, fine dice

3 onions, fine dice

3 garlic cloves, chopped

3 tablespoons nonfat sour cream

3 egg whites
Salt and pepper to taste

Sear venison in hot canola oil or in a pan until rare. Season with pepper and rest.

In a large mixing bowl combine crab meat, red bell pepper, green bell pepper, yellow bell pepper, fennel, and onion.

In a small mixing bowl combine nonfat sour cream, egg white, garlic, salt, and pepper.

Combine sour cream mixture with crab meat.

Place venison on sheet pan and crown with crab-meat mixture. Warm the medallions under the broiler to serving temperature—about 3 to 4 minutes. Crab meat should begin to brown slightly.

Nutrition pyramid servings: 3 meat, .5 vegetable

If you are feeling adventurous try this unique recipe for Crab-Crowned Venison Medallions. If you do not have a local source of venison, there are many resources on the Web.

Santa Clara County

www.californiacoastalwines.com
www.santaclarachamber.org
www.scvwga.com

Leaving the Gold Country we're going to head on back toward the California coast. Follow highways 108 and 120 west onto 580, then south on 680 to the bottom of the San Francisco Bay, and turn west through the city of San Jose. At this point you will take Highway 17 to our next stop, the town of Los Gatos. While these days Santa Clara County is primarily known as the home of Silicon Valley, its billionaires, and Stanford University, in the early 1900s there were over one hundred wineries here. Among the wineries that continue to thrive despite urban expansion is Mirassou, whose wine-growing family dates back to the 1800s, giving them the distinction of being America's oldest winemaking family.

In the beautiful town of Los Gatos, which lies between Silicon Valley and the Santa Cruz Mountains, we are going to visit Manresa Restaurant.

Chef and owner David Kinch graduated from Johnson and Wales Culinary Academy in Rhode Island. He worked at three renowned restaurants in Europe, as executive chef at both Ernie's and Silks in San Francisco and for four years at the esteemed Quilted Giraffe in New York City. Kinch earned national recognition for his artisanal approach to contemporary cuisine at Restaurant Sent Sovi in Saratoga, California. *Zagat Guides* writes that "David Kinch has raised the bar for restaurants in the South Bay" with "boldly flavored Catalan-accented New French dishes that you dream about for days."

Manresa Restaurant
320 Village Lane
Los Gatos, CA 95030
(408) 354-4330
www.manresarestaurant.com

Recipe from the Manresa Restaurant
by Chef David Kinch

Strawberry Gazpacho

Serves 6

1 pound, 4 ounces strawberries, hulled and lightly crushed
4 ounces white onions, thinly sliced
4 ounces red bell peppers, thinly sliced
5 ounces cucumber, peeled, seeded, thinly sliced
Half clove garlic, crushed
¼ cup of tarragon leaves (5 grams)
¼ cup balsamic vinegar
¼ cup extra-virgin olive oil

For garnish:
Strawberries, hulled and finely diced
Chives, finely minced
Red bell pepper, finely diced
English cucumber, peeled, seeded, finely diced

2 tablespoons almond oil
Chervil sprigs

Place all ingredients in a bowl, mix well, cover with plastic wrap, and refrigerate overnight. The next day puree in a blender and season with salt and pepper.

If it is too thick, you can thin with water. Allow to thoroughly chill.

For the garnish, gently toss all the diced vegetables and fruit and toss lightly with almond oil. Mound in the center of a soup plate and top with some chervil sprigs. Pour the gazpacho over the garnish tableside.

Nutrition pyramid servings: .5 vegetable, .5 fruit, 2 oil

This beautiful, light, delicious Strawberry Gazpacho makes the perfect California Wine Country Diet soup for a warm day out on your deck. It may be all you want or need for lunch or dinner.

Also in Los Gatos you will find the California Cafe which includes a wide range of California-style cuisine under the direction of Chef Simon Hernandez. In the relaxing atmosphere of the California Cafe, who can resist the seasonal food menu or the extensive "Liquid Therapy" menu with items such as "Pampered Pear Martini" and "Siesta Sangria."

California Cafe
Old Town 50 University Avenue, Suite 260
Los Gatos, CA 95030
(408) 354-8118
www.CaliforniaCafe.com

Recipe from the California Cafe

by Chef Simon Hernandez

Angel Hair Pasta and Prawns

Serves 4
2/3 pound jumbo prawns
2 fresh tomatoes, diced, or 1 8-ounce can

1½ ounces tomato juice
½ tablespoon garlic, peeled and chopped
1 tablespoon basil, julienned
1 tablespoon extra-virgin olive oil
¼ pound angel hair pasta (amount to your taste)

Cook pasta in boiling water for 4 minutes, then drain.

Heat a pan, spray with olive oil to cover, and add 1 tablespoon of olive oil. Sauté shrimp and garlic until lightly cooked. Add other ingredients until they are cooked, and then add the pasta to reheat. Serve on plate with basil to garnish.

Nutrition pyramid servings: 1 grain, .5 vegetable, 2 protein, .75 oil

This delicious pasta is easy to prepare on any night of the week. You can enjoy it is, as it is or try adding other wine country ingredients such as artichoke hearts, black olives, or feta cheese. A green salad, some grilled bread, and you have dinner.

Monterey County

www.californiacoastalwines.com
www.montereyinfo.org
www.montereywines.org

From Los Gatos it's time to head south again on Highway 101. After leaving San Jose you will be traveling through southern Santa Clara County and the town of Gilroy, which is known as the "Garlic Capital of the World." It is said that 90 percent of America's garlic is grown here. The annual garlic festival is a highlight of the summer. The area has an abundance of wineries that are within easy access of Highway 101. See the above Web sites for directions.

At Salinas you will continue west on Route 68 to the town of Monterey. Though this area is best known for tourism, John Steinbeck novels, and golf tournaments, it is in fact one of the major grape-growing areas of California. Wine production began in the 1960s, when vintners from the north began looking for more land as the Bay Area population expanded. A study of California wine-growing regions was published at this time that rated Monterey County's climate as "equivalent to not only Napa and Sonoma but also France's famous wine regions of Burgundy and Bordeaux." The cooling fog, which streams from the Pacific Ocean across the Monterey Bay, makes this an ideal area in which to plant white varietals.

Fifty percent of the county's grape production is Chardonnay. Other award-winning varietals that flourish in the area's many microclimates include Merlot, Cabernet Sauvignon, Pinot Noir, Riesling, and Syrah. There are over fifty wineries in the Salinas and Carmel valleys to visit, as well as tasting rooms in Monterey and Carmel.

When you're not wine tasting, there are limitless other things to do: Visit Cannery Row (made famous by John Steinbeck), the world-class Monterey Aquarium, art galleries, and gift shops, to name a few.

Right past Monterey is the town of Pacific Grove and the Fandango Restaurant, located in a charming old house. The fun-loving atmosphere here hasn't faded since Pierre and Marietta Bain first purchased it in 1986 from its original owner. Although Bain was then the manager of Club XIX at The Lodge at Pebble Beach, something "struck a chord with him" when he visited the restaurant for the first time. (In fact, Pierre Bain's family has operated the Grand Hôtel Bain at Comp-sur-Artuby in the south of France since 1737.) A book about the restaurant was published in 1993 entitled *Fandango, The Story of Two Guys Who Wanted to Own a Restaurant (Fortunately One Knew What He Was Doing)*. Fandango features Mediterranean and European-style cuisine and is the winner of many awards including the Wine Spectator Best of Award of Excellence.

Fandango Restaurant
223 17th Street
Pacific Grove, CA 93950
(831) 372-3456
www.fandangorestaurant.com

Recipes from the Fandango Restaurant

by Owners Pierre and Marietta Bain

Giant Sea Scallops Fandango

Serves 1 (Multiply recipe by the number of desired servings)
5 giant sea scallops (10 to the pound)
Flour to cover
1 tablespoon butter
1 shallot, chopped
1 ounce white wine
¼ lemon, squeezed
½ ounce demi-glace (optional)
Parsley
Salt and pepper to taste after cooked

Dredge scallops in flour and sauté in butter and shallots. When almost cooked, add white wine and lemon juice, sauté all briefly, then remove scallops from pan.

Continue to reduce the liquid, and add the capers and demi-glace. Pour this reduced mixture over the sautéed scallops.

Sprinkle with parsley.

Nutrition pyramid servings: 2.5 meat, 100 pleasure food calories for the butter

Chef's wine suggestion: Gewurztraminer or Pinot Blanc

This superb yet easy way to prepare sea scallops makes for a delightful focus of a dinner. The original recipe calls for 4 tablespoons of butter. We reduced it to 1 tablespoon and it still works. You will need to use 100 of your pleasure food calories to prepare this dish with butter. It is well worth it. Demi-glace is a rich espagnole sauce that uses beef stock slowly cooked with sherry or Madeira wine until it is reduced by half. This dish is also delicious without the demi-glace.

Lamb Shanks

Serves 10

2 lamb shanks (approximately 1 pound each)

½ cup flour

¼ cup olive oil

Salt and pepper, a dash each

1 tablespoon butter

2 shallots, finely chopped

1 clove garlic (small) finely chopped

2 teaspoons yellow onion, finely chopped

¼ teaspoon thyme leaves, whole

¼ teaspoon rosemary leaves

½ cup white wine

½ cup red wine

½ teaspoon basil, crushed

1½ cup lamb stock (chicken stock can be substituted if necessary)

1 carrot (large) quartered and cut in 2-inch chunks

1 turnip (large), cut in half and then quartered

8 mushrooms, quartered

¼ cup peas, fresh or frozen

8 pearl onions

2 tablespoons cognac (brandy may be substituted)

Trim fat, and remove fell (thin outer skin) from lamb shanks; salt and pepper shanks and dredge in flour.

Heat olive oil in medium-sized skillet until it smokes; add lamb shanks and brown.

In a separate ovenproof skillet, melt butter and add shallots, garlic, onion, rosemary, and thyme; simmer mixture, but do not let butter brown.

When onions are transparent, add lamb shanks, red and white wines, and let simmer, covered, for 30 minutes, turning the shanks over after the first 15 minutes to cook evenly.

Preheat oven to 350 degrees. Add 1½ cups lamb stock, stir in a dash of basil, and bake covered, for 1 hour or until tender. Check the shanks every 15 minutes and baste with juices. Add additional lamb stock if necessary, so that the shanks do not dry out.

After the first 30 minutes, add carrots, turnips, mushrooms, and peas. Continue to bake. Before serving, stir in cognac, and salt and pepper to taste.

Nutrition pyramid servings: 1 grain, 3 meat (3 ounces of lamb), 1.5 vegetable, 1.5 oil, 25 pleasure food calories for the butter

Chef's wine suggestion: Sangiovese or Cabernet Sauvignon

Note from the chefs: "We season our lamb stock with celery, onions, carrots, leeks, garlic, rosemary, thyme, bay leaves, and freshly ground black pepper."

This is a rich and special dinner to prepare for a cold winter's night. Sip Sangiovese by the fire as you wait for your lamb shanks to cook. The original restaurant recipe calls for ½ cup of olive oil for browning the lamb shanks. We have reduced the amount to ¼ cup to reduce the amount of oil servings. It helps to use an oil spray to cover the skillet. The chefs suggest serving this with boiled new potatoes.

When you leave Pacific Grove, be sure to take the world-famous Seventeen Mile Drive, which takes you south through some of the most stunning scenery on the planet. There are six golf courses along the way including Pebble Beach and Monterey Peninsula, scene of the AT&T Pro-Am golf tournament. At the end of the Seventeen Mile Drive, you will come to Carmel, also known as Carmel-by-the-Sea, which was founded by a group of artists and writers as a retreat in 1904. The town of Carmel has managed to retain much of its charm despite the abundance of tourists who visit its shops, galleries, and restaurants.

In the heart of Carmel is Bouchée Restaurant, Wine Bar, and Bouchée Wine Merchants opened by David and Kathleen Fink in 2002.

David Fink has been associated with some of Northern California's finest luxury resorts, hotels, and restaurants, most recently as general manager of The Lodge at Pebble Beach. He says that they wanted the restaurant to be "very comfortable and affordable with delicious food and a very wonderful wine list." Kathleen Fink explains that the translation of *bouchée* is "mouthful. We think of it as delicious mouthfuls to be served in a setting of simple elegance."

The executive chef of Bouchée Restaurant, Walter Manzke, first met David Fink at the Carmel Highlands Masters of Food and Wine event, of which Fink is a founder. It was then that Manzke first fell in love with the Carmel area. Manzke has trained in some of the most renowned kitchens in America and Europe. For six years prior to moving to Carmel he worked at the famed Patina Restaurant and at hundreds of spectacular dinners around the world with long-time mentor Joachim Splichal. For the menu at Bouchée, Manzke organizes dishes according to their origins: Garden, Ocean, Farm, and Forest—seasonally. He says that all the dishes are designed to complement and be complemented by good wine. And he has the restaurant's 4,000-bottle wine cellar to choose from.

Bouchée Restaurant
Mission (Between Ocean and 7th)
Carmel By the Sea, CA 93921
(831) 626-7882
www.boucheecarmel.com

Recipe from Bouchée Restaurant

by Executive Chef Walter Manzke

Heirloom Tomatoes with Buratta Cheese, Watermelon and White Balsamic Granité

Serves 8

2 pounds Heirloom tomatoes (select tomatoes of different sizes, shapes and colors)

1 pound of Buratta cheese

1 slice of watermelon, cut in ½-inch cubes

6 leaves of fresh basil, torn into medium pieces

2 tablespoons extra-virgin olive oil

White balsamic granité (see below)

Sea salt and freshly-ground pepper to taste

Slice the large tomatoes into ¼-inch thick slices. Halve or quarter the smaller tomatoes.

In the center of a medium-size round plate, place 1 slice of room temperature Buratta cheese and a slice of tomato. Working outward alternate cheese and tomato slices in a spiral. Randomly arrange the smaller tomato quarters and halves between and around the spiral. Season with sea salt and freshly ground pepper.

Place 5 or 6 cubes of watermelon and the torn basil leaves over the tomatoes. Drizzle with extra-virgin olive oil.

Shave the frozen balsamic granité with a fork and scatter over the tomatoes.

Serve immediately before the granité melts.

White Balsamic Granité
½ cup white balsamic vinegar
2 tablespoons mineral water

Mix both ingredients in a small bowl and freeze.

Nutrition pyramid servings: 1 vegetable, .75 fruit, .5 oil, 1 dairy and 80 pleasure food calories for the cheese.

This is a beautiful salad that you will want to make when both Heirloom tomatoes and watermelon are at the height of their ripeness in late summer. *Granité* is French for ice.

Olive Oil Poached Salmon, Braised Baby Artichokes, Artichoke Purée and Sauvignon Blanc Sauce

Serves 8
2 lemons
4 medium artichokes
½ onion
1 stalk of celery
2 tablespoons extra-virgin olive oil
2 cloves of garlic, peeled and halved
1 cup Sauvignon Blanc
2 sprigs fresh thyme
4 6-ounce salmon filets with the skin on

Sea salt
8–10 cups olive oil
1 cup chicken stock
½ teaspoon sherry vinegar
1 cup reduced chicken stock (reduce regular by half)
2 tablespoons extra-virgin olive oil
White pepper to taste
2 tablespoons parsley, chopped

Squeeze the juice of 1 lemon into bowl of cold water. Clean artichokes (remove tough outer leaves, cut off tops, trim outer heart, and remove choke). Cut in half and then thirds, and place them in the lemon-water.

Slice onion and celery into thick chunks. In a stainless steel pot, heat 2 tablespoons olive oil, and sweat onions, celery, and garlic. Add artichokes, the juice of 1 lemon, wine, and the thyme sprigs. Lightly cover and simmer until the artichokes are cooked. (If the pan starts to dry out before artichokes are done, add hot water in small amounts.) Remove and discard the onions, garlic, celery, and thyme. Season with sea salt.

Season salmon with sea salt. Fill a saucepan large enough to hold all the salmon in a single layer without touching with the olive oil. Heat to 150 degrees. Submerge the salmon in the oil and cook for about 20 minutes. Don't let salmon get hotter than 150 degrees.

Place 1/3 of the artichokes in a small saucepan. Cover with 1 cup chicken stock, 1 tablespoon extra-virgin olive oil, and vinegar. Simmer for about 10 minutes until falling-apart tender. Remove the artichokes, season with salt and pepper, and purée in a blender until thick and smooth.

Cook the rest of the artichokes with the remaining (now reduced) chicken stock until the stock is again reduced by half. Away from the heat, mix in 1 tablespoon extra-virgin olive oil. Season with sea salt, freshly ground white pepper, and chopped parsley.

Remove salmon from oil bath. Place skin side down in a hot skillet for 2 minutes to crisp the skin and finish the cooking.

Place a spoonful of purée in the center of a large flat bowl for each serving. Place salmon skin side up on the purée, and spoon the artichokes with their sauce around the salmon.

Nutrition pyramid servings: 1.5 vegetable, 2 oil, 3 meat

This heavenly dish is a favorite with customers at Bouchée. I can't remember ever having eaten salmon this moist and tender. I have been assured by several chefs that the salmon does not absorb the poaching oil which is why we have not counted it in the nutritional breakdown. We have reduced the serving size from 6 ounces of salmon to 3 ounces.

San Luis Obispo County

www.escalen.org
www.sanluisobispocounty.com
www.pasowine.com

Heading south from Carmel you have two routes to choose from: Route 1, the coastal highway, and the inland route of Highway 101. If you choose Highway 1, you will be driving through the majestic scenery of Big Sur with redwood forests on your left and the Pacific Ocean crashing on your right. You can camp in Los Padres National Forest, and you can stop for a massage and bath in the mineral hot springs perched on a rocky ledge fifty feet above the ocean at the Esalen Institute. Farther down the road you can visit Hearst Castle at San Simeon, which was built by newspaper publisher William Randolph Hearst. In this castle of 165 rooms overlooking the Pacific Ocean, he entertained the Hollywood elite from the 1920s until the late 1940s. If your choice is Highway 101, there is nothing nearly as exciting to see but you will arrive earlier in Paso Robles and will not have to endure the twists and turns of the winding coastal highway.

Most of the grape growing in San Luis Obispo County began in the 1970s, when growers from the Napa Valley and Sonoma discovered that the conditions were ideal for growing premium wine grapes. Wineries today are springing up everywhere, and it is said that San Luis Obispo and Santa Barbara counties together make up the fastest growing wine area in the United States. Unlike the rest of the county, grape growing in the Paso Robles area dates back to the 1800s. Award-winning Zinfandel, Pinot Noir, Cabernet, Chardonnay, and Sauvignon Blanc are all grown in the Paso Robles area of San Luis Obispo County.

Our next stop is at the Justin Vineyards and Winery in Paso Robles. In 1981, Justin and Deborah Baldwin bought seventy-two acres and began to produce small lots of wine by 1987. Their wines have gone on to win many awards. On the grounds of the winery are not only a tasting room but a bed and breakfast and a restaurant. At the JUST Inn you can relax in luxury suites furnished in fine European tradition and then stroll in the English gardens. Nightly dinners and weekend lunches are served in Deborah's Room restaurant. Prepared by Executive Chef Ryan Swarthout, the menus emphasize seasonal, fresh ingredients along with Justin select wines.

Gourmet Magazine calls the food "Seamless!" and *Wine Spectator* has said, "Justin Vineyards and Winery are not to be missed and are in a class by themselves."

Justin Vineyards & Winery
JUST Inn/Deborah's Room
11680 Chimney Rock Road
Paso Robles, CA 93446
(805) 237-4149 (800) 238-0049
www.justinwine.com

Recipes from Deborah's Room at Justin Vineyards & Winery

by Executive Chef Ryan Swarthout

Heirloom Tomato Gazpacho

Serves 12

1 piece of good-quality bread, without the crust (about 2–3 inches long)
1 garlic clove, peeled
1 whole shallot, peeled
2 teaspoons salt
1 teaspoon sugar
2 tablespoons balsamic vinegar
½ teaspoon ground cumin
2 pounds ripe Heirloom tomatoes, cored and quartered
¾ cup extra-virgin olive oil

Cut the crust-less bread into large cubes. Soak bread cubes in about

½ cup of water for 1 minute, then squeeze dry and discard water. In a food processor, combine bread, garlic, shallots, salt, sugar, vinegar, cumin, and half of the tomatoes. Puree. While the food processor is running, add the remaining tomatoes and continue pureeing. Slowly drizzle the extra-virgin olive oil in a steady stream and blend until smooth (about 1 minute). Strain soup through a fine sieve into a bowl. Push solids through the strainer firmly and discard any left over. Taste for seasoning, and adjust with salt and pepper if necessary. Serve soup immediately or refrigerate for later.

Optional garnish: Chive oil and crispy basil leaves (recipes follow).

Chive Oil

1 cup olive oil
1 bunch of chives

Place all of the ingredients in a blender and puree for 1 minute. Pour oil through a fine strainer. Drizzle on top of soup.

Crispy Basil

3 tablespoons olive oil
4 basil leaves

Heat oil over medium heat. Fry the basil for 30 seconds on both sides. Place on a paper towel to drain the oil. Garnish the soup with the crispy basil right before serving.

Nutrition pyramid servings: .5 vegetable, 2.5 oil

Chef's wine suggestion: Justin Chardonnay

Chef Swarthout says, "This is a perfect warm-weather soup with exquisite flavor and depth. Choose top quality Heirloom tomatoes that are ripe and bursting with flavor. They're easy to find during August and September at local farmers' markets and are essential to the flavor development of the gazpacho. Be sure to serve this soup with Justin Chardonnay —the light touch of oak and balanced acidity make it a perfect foil for the velvety-smooth depth of the gazpacho."

I'm sure most readers are wishing that they could enjoy this Heirloom Tomato Gazpacho on the patio of Deborah's Room overlooking the vineyards on a warm summer's day. Even if you can't make it there, I guarantee that you will enjoy this gazpacho right on your own patio. The original restaurant recipe calls for 1½ cups of olive oil which we have reduced to ¾ cup.

Santa Barbara County

www.californiacoastalwines.com
www.sbcountywines.com
www.santabarbaraca.com

Leaving Paso Robles on Highway 101, we will travel back toward the ocean at San Luis Obispo and then inland through Santa Maria and into the Santa Inez Valley. There are at least five dozen wineries in Santa Barbara County, most in the Santa Ynez and Santa Maria valleys. The better known wineries include Fess Parker, Gainey, and Firestone, along with many small wineries. This is one of the state's growing wine areas, with new wineries opening up at a rapid rate. There's lots of land that is drawing adventurous people who want to try their hand at growing grapes. The multitude of microclimates makes this an area that is good for growing just about every varietal.

The Santa Inez Valley has gained world attention with the release in the fall of 2004 of the movie *Sideways*, which won a Golden Globe for best comedy and was nominated for five Oscars. The story about two friends who set out on a wine-tasting tour of the Santa Inez Valley before one gets married has sparked great interest in this California wine country area that often is overshadowed by Northern California's wine country. Thousands of maps have been published and downloaded by tourists wanting to retrace the steps of the two wine-drinking friends, Miles and Jack, as they toured the area's tasting rooms and restaurants.

In *Sideways,* the main characters enjoy a leisurely meal accompanied by Miles' favorite wine, Pinot Noir, in the warm, inviting atmosphere of the Los Olivos Café. Serving California–Mediterranean cuisine, the Los Olivos

Café was already an acclaimed restaurant in the area when the movie brought them an incredible surge of business.

The Café's owner, Sam Marmorstein, moved to the town of Los Olivos in 1995 from Los Angeles, where he was a stockbroker. He bought land to establish a winery and a former downtown deli that he transformed into the Los Olivos Café. In 2001, he opened The Wine Merchant, tasting bar, deli, and gift shop next door. Gourmet products such as the Los Olivos Café Bread Dipping Oil and Olive Tapenade are sold in the store and online worldwide.

Executive Chef Nat Ely was born in Hawaii and began his career in Seattle, where he advanced to lead chef at Festivities Bistro and then Place Pigale. Prior to coming to the Los Olivos Café, he was sous-chef at Birnham Wood Country Club in Montecito and Emilio's Ristorante in Santa Barbara. He creates unique hand-crafted dishes using the freshest seasonal ingredients. The café features a special "Sideways Menu" including, of course, a glass of Pinot Noir.

Los Olivos Café
2879 Grand Avenue,
Los Olivos, CA 93441
(805) 688-7265
www.losolivoscafe.com

Recipes from the Los Olivos Café

by Executive Chef Nat Ely

Pan-Fried Willapa Bay Oysters with Hearts of Palm, Red Endive, and Scallions Salad with Buttermilk Vinaigrette

Serves 2-4

Pan Fried Willapa Bay Oysters
16 choice oysters, shucked (use scrutiny to ensure quality)
1½ cups white flour

2 teaspoons ground sea salt

1 teaspoon ground black pepper

2 teaspoons chili powder (can add cayenne for more heat if you
   desire)

Mix the flour and spices and spread on a baking sheet or large plate.

Roll oysters in flour mixture and fry (until light brown on both sides) in a medium-hot pan.

Buttermilk Vinaigrette
1 cup buttermilk

3 tablespoons lemon juice

¼ cup pure olive oil

½ teaspoon salt

Hearts of Palm, Red Endive, and Scallions Salad
8 to12 ounces fresh or canned hearts of palm, sliced on a bias

4 heads of red or white Belgian endive, julienned

2 scallions, julienned

In a medium bowl, add salad items and ¼ cup of buttermilk vinaigrette. Toss until coated.

Arrange salad mixture on serving plates, spoon remaining buttermilk vinaigrette onto plate, and set crispy oysters on plate. Snipped chives make a nice addition for garnish.

Nutrition pyramid servings: 1 serving = 4 oysters and 2 cups of salad. Oysters: .5 grain, 2 protein; salad: 2 vegetable; vinaigrette: 1 oil

Chef's wine suggestion: Chenin Blanc or Chardonnay.

This delicious salad is easy enough to make on a weeknight and special enough for any guest. Make sure you pat the oysters dry before rolling them in the flour and that the pan is hot enough. Served with some grilled bread, it is enough for a whole meal. If oysters are not in season, you can also make this with good-quality jarred oysters.

Café Panzanella Salad

Serves 4

3 cups hand-cut and oven-dried Artisan bread croutons, medium diced

4 cups vine-ripened tomatoes, medium diced

1 cup cucumber, peeled and seeded, medium diced

¼ cup red onion, small diced

¼ cup pistachios, toasted and crushed

¼ cup Gorgonzola, crumbled

¼ cup basil, julienned

Dressing

1½ cup pure olive oil

½ cup balsamic vinegar

2 tablespoons Dijon mustard

2 tablespoons julienned basil

Salt and pepper to taste

Place all ingredients for the dressing, except the oil, in a blender or food processor. Blend on low and slowly stream in olive oil, and reserve.

Place the croutons, tomatoes, cucumbers, and onion in a medium mixing bowl and coat with amount of dressing to your liking. Spoon mixture evenly onto selected plates. Evenly spread Gorgonzola, pistachios, and julienned basil on top of salad. Garnish with basil tops and enjoy.

Nutrition pyramid servings: Salad: 1 grain, 2 vegetable, 1 nut, 1 dairy

Dressing: 1 tablespoon = 2 oil

Chef's wine suggestion: Sangiovese, Barbera, or Pinot Noir

Nat Ely says, "This dish is our representation of an Italian summer classic."

These two salads by Chef Ely include nutritious ingredients in delicious and easy recipes. That is why we have chosen both salads to be part of our initial three-week meal plans.

We are now coming to our last stop on the tour of California's different wine areas. Our tour, which began in the magnificent redwoods of Humboldt County, now ends in the equally breathtaking, though very different, coastal town of Santa Barbara. In the heart of downtown is bouchon santa barbara restaurant, which opened on Bastille Day in 1998. In French *bouchon* means "wine cork," and Mitchell Sjerven, the owner, is an enthusiastic supporter of the rapidly expanding Santa Barbara area's wine industry.

The restaurant's wine list includes over forty Central Coast wines that you can order by the glass. The atmosphere of the restaurant reflects fine dining that is served at a relaxed and leisurely pace. The food is based on the philosophy of using ingredients that are as fresh and local as possible. *Bon Appétit Magazine* says, "Bouchon offers an education of the region's agriculture and viniculture." *The San Francisco Chronicle* described bouchon as "Perfect."

Having worked in the restaurant industry for twenty years, it seems that Mitchell Sjerven is always taking on new challenges. He is president of the board of directors for the Santa Barbara Conference and Visitors Bureau & Film Commission and was recently selected to sit on the California Restaurant Advisory Committee. In 2000, bouchon santa barbara was selected by the State of California to be the exclusive caterer for the IMAX film *Adventures in Wild California*. He and Josh Brown brought California cuisine to thousands of moviegoers in twenty international cities.

Chef Josh Brown graduated from the culinary program at Santa Barbara City College and went on to work for some of the better restaurants in Santa Barbara. He has been chef at bouchon since 2003 and says that one of his favorite things about the restaurant is the open cooking line that allows guests to come up to the window and let him know how they enjoyed the dinner. Brown has been on the television show "Cooking with Laura McIntosh" and on "Food Nation with Bobby Flay."

The Roasted Carrot Soup and the English Pea & Toasted Cumin Salad dishes have special meaning as they are the recipes that bouchon santa barbara cooked for the 13th Annual James Beard Journalism Awards Dinner in May of 2005. The theme of the dinner was "Boston and Santa Barbara Chefs' Tribute to Julia Child." They were asked to prepare a first course and chose the Roasted Carrot Soup that "Julia loved." The soup was served on a long, rectangular plate with the soup on one half and the pea salad on the other. Mr. Sjerven said, "The idea was to present the two philosophies behind market cooking: taking wonderful, organic ingredients and cooking a delicious dish (the soup) and taking beautiful, organic flavors and leaving them to shine more or less 'on their own' (the spring pea salad)."

I asked Mr. Sjerven to talk a little about when Julia Child visited bouchon santa barbara. He said, ""Julia Child was a wonderful personality to have in the restaurant, of course. But beyond the stargazing by happy clientele was a warmth and familiarity that made everyone comfortable. She was not interested in fad or fashion but rather solid, flavorful food—what we now call 'comfort food' but she simply called 'good, simple cooking.' She did enjoy keeping up with the burgeoning local wine scene, though, preferring full-bodied Syrah with our braised short ribs and crisp, lesser-oaked Chardonnay with roasted chicken."

bouchon santa barbara
9 West Victoria Street
Santa Barbara, CA 93101
(805) 730 - 1160
www.bouchonsantabarbara.com

Recipes from bouchon santa barbara:

by Chef Josh Brown

Roasted Carrot Soup

Serves 4 first-course size portions
5 pounds farmers' market carrots, peeled and diced
2 yellow onions, medium, diced
3 stalks celery, diced
4 cloves garlic, crushed
1 leek, white part only, chopped
2 tablespoons ginger, peeled and minced
3 tablespoons olive oil

In a heavy-bottomed pot, heat olive oil over high heat until almost smoking. Carefully add onions, celery, garlic, leek, and ginger, then stir. Lower heat to medium and slowly cook vegetables for 5 to 8 minutes, until the onion becomes translucent but not browned.

Add chopped carrots, cooking another 3 minutes. Add 2 quarts water and herbs and bring heat back to high. Bring to boil then reduce heat to simmer until carrots are tender and cooked through. Add or reduce water for thinner or thicker soup. Remove from heat and let cool slightly.

Ladle soup into blender and puree on high until smooth. (You may need to do this in batches depending on the size of your blender or food processor.)

Put soup back in pot over medium heat and season to taste, warming to serve.

Nutrition pyramid servings: 8.5 vegetable, 2 oil

Chef's wine suggestion: "For a lighter white wine accompaniment, yet still crisp and dry, try Babcock Vineyards Pinot Grigio."

This is a delicious, healthy, and easy to prepare carrot soup. The ginger gives it zing. For a wonderful soup and salad combo, see the English Pea & Toasted Cumin Salad recipe below.

English Pea & Toasted Cumin Salad

6 small first-course size portions
2 cups English peas, shelled
1 teaspoon shallots, minced
1 teaspoon mint, chopped
1 cup carrots, julienned
1 tablespoon cumin seed, toasted and cracked
¼ cup sherry vinaigrette
Salt and pepper to taste

Sherry Vinaigrette
1 cup extra-virgin olive oil
1/3 cup sherry vinegar

1 teaspoon chopped fresh thyme and
1 teaspoon Dijon mustard

In a large pot bring 3 quarts of water and 2 tablespoons salt to boil. Fill a large bowl with ice and water and place within reach in your work area.

Blanch shelled English peas in boiling water for 2 to 3 minutes. You are looking for a still firm pea. Avoid overcooking. Remove peas from water with slotted spoon or similar utensil and put in ice bath. Repeat with carrots, blanching for 1 to 2 minutes and then placing them in the ice bath.

Once cool, strain and place peas and carrots in medium bowl and toss with shallots, garlic, and cumin and season to taste with salt and pepper.

Dress with sherry vinaigrette.

Nutrition pyramid servings: 1 vegetable, 1.5 oil

Chef's wine suggestion: "When choosing a wine, the refreshing 'garden flavors' of this salad lend themselves well to a Sauvignon Blanc, such as the one from Fiddlehead Cellars. Winemaker Kathy Joseph makes one she calls Gooseberry that is phenomenal with spring market flavors."

A beautiful and delicious companion to the Roasted Carrot Soup or just alone with crusty bread.

Grilled Rosemary-Skewered Scallops

12 appetizers (2 scallops per skewer) or 6 entrees (4 scallops per skewer)
24 each U-10 size scallops (jumbo) dry-pack fresh
1 ounce grapeseed oil
2 limes
Salt and pepper to taste
Rosemary twigs

Skewer scallops with rosemary twigs and brush with grapeseed oil (so they don't stick to the grill) and fresh lime juice. Do not allow scallops and lime juice to touch until just before grilling, or you will end up with ceviche!

Grill on high but for a very short time. Grill temperatures vary so watch them; overcooked scallops are rubbery, whereas medium-rare scallops are heaven. A minute for the first side and 30 seconds for the other side is a good approximation. Try one skewer first; check doneness before cooking the rest of your skewers. Scallops should just be getting firm, not hard, when you pull them from the grill. Once off the grill keep in mind they'll continue to cook for several seconds.

Nutrition pyramid servings: Appetizer portion: 1 meat, .5 oil; Entree portion: 2 meat, 1 oil

Chef's wine suggestions: "I prefer a very crisp white, like Westerly Sauvignon Blanc or Brander Vineyards 'Au Naturel.' Alternatively, a brighter, light-bodied Pinot Noir works great too if you are already in the red-zone by the time you serve the scallops. Since they are grilled with a rosemary skewer, a smoky, earthy Pinot works well. Try Au Bon Climat or Hitching Post Bien Nacido."

This simple preparation of scallops allows their natural flavor to come through. Try the entree at night and make extra for a salad the next day. For a lighter meal or appetizer, serve over greens with a citrus dressing. For a delicious entree, serve over asparagus risotto and crispy pancetta garnish.

Smoked Pacific Albacore with White Bean Puree, Pesto, and Oven Roasted Tomatoes

Serves 8
2 pounds smoked albacore
White bean puree (see recipe below)
Pesto (see recipe below)
Roasted tomatoes (see recipe below)
Herbs de Provence
Coarse salt

White Bean Puree
2 cups dried white beans, soaked in 2 quarts water overnight
½ cup white onion, diced

3 cloves of garlic
1 tablespoon olive oil
Salt and pepper to taste
1 tablespoon butter (optional)

Cook soaked beans in simmering pot of water with onion and garlic until soft. Strain and let moisture drain out in a warm place. Blend in food processor until smooth, slowly adding butter and olive oil. Season to taste and keep warm until ready to serve.

Pesto
2 cups fresh basil, tightly packed
Juice of 1 lemon
4 garlic cloves
2 tablespoons Parmigiano cheese, grated
2 cups olive oil

In food processor blend garlic, lemon juice, and herbs. While operating processor at slow speed, add in olive oil until the herbs are minced and the mixture is slightly chunky. Add Parmigiano and season to taste.

Oven-Roasted Tomatoes
10 Roma tomatoes, sliced in half lengthwise
2 tablespoons Italian parsley
Olive oil or oil spray

Sprinkle garlic and parsley on top of halved Roma tomatoes. Drizzle with small amount of olive oil, place in oven, and let roast on a low oven setting for approximately 5 hours.

If you are smoking the fish yourself, do so ever so lightly, preferably with oak, being careful not to over smoke and thus overpower the albacore flavor. Coat exterior of albacore with herbs de Provence and coarse salt mixture. On very hot skillet, in 3 tablespoons of oil, sear fish by turning 3 times to *crust* the exterior of the fish and yet keep the light purple center rare.

Place mound of white bean purée just off-center on the plate, slice albacore and fan slices out around white bean puree. Add roasted tomatoes and drizzle pesto all around the plate.

Serve with sautéed greens, asparagus, or haricots verts (green beans).

Nutrition pyramid servings: Fish, beans, tomatoes: 1 vegetable, .5 oil, 5 meat (includes 1 serving beans); Pesto: 1 tablespoon = 2 oil

Chef's wine suggestions: "For the Sauvignon Blanc lover this dish presents wonderful possibilities. With an abundance of herbs, veggies, and fish the Brander 'Au Naturel' is a perfect match. Lots of acid, no oak, and ready to take on this dish with zest. Those who go straight to Pinot Noir with fish these days, however, won't be disappointed. Albacore is particularly well-suited to the earthy strains of Santa Barbara County Pinots. Try the Fiddlehead Cellars, Clos Pepe Estate, or Melville Vineyards for some wonderful wines that have an excellent balance of earthiness and fruit without being too ripe."

You have a wonderful dining experience waiting for you with this dish. There are actually four recipes within this, all of which can be used in combination with other foods. The original restaurant recipe for this served four. We have increased this to eight servings to accommodate the lower calorie plans. If you want a larger serving, you can use your pleasure food calories for the additional meat and beans. Herbs de Provence is a melding of traditional herbs from the southeast part of France. It is available at gourmet shops and fine grocery stores.

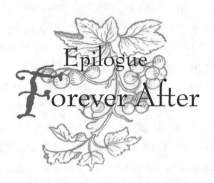

Epilogue
Forever After

"Moderation, small helpings, and a great variety of foods is a great precept...But most of all...have a good time!"
—*Julia Child, when asked to sum up her philosophy on eating*

I hope that you have enjoyed your tour of the California wine country and that you have begun to prepare some of these wonderful restaurant recipes yourself. You have come a long way since John Ash first talked in the Foreword about the importance of eating wholesome, fresh, seasonal food and the enjoyable and healthy place wine can have in our lives. Over the course of this book, you have become familiar with the six aspects of the Wheel of Weight-Management and come to understand the vital role each aspect of the Wheel plays in supporting a healthy lifestyle. Whatever your activity level was at the beginning of this program, you are probably more active now. Through the California Wine Country Diet Meal Plans, you have begun to establish a new way of eating that meets your nutritional needs and fulfills the desires of both your conscious and your basic selves. You have begun to practice the art of Conscious Indulgence so that you can also continue to enjoy the foods and beverages that give you the most pleasure.

It is time now to look ahead to some of the challenges you may face as you continue on the program and to consider effective strategies for dealing with them. It seems to me that diets are much like marriages. There is the initial search for "the right one," then comes the infatuation when you think you have found it, and then the honeymoon that sustains the glow. But once you return to "normal" life, the real work begins. You face the realities of living day to day, or growing and changing, of dealing with different situations and new circumstances. In a marriage those first reality checks might appear soon after the honeymoon glow begins to fade and you see more clearly the humanness of your beloved. You do not fall out of love or lose your commitment. You adapt.

A diet or lifestyle change can follow this same pattern, with the honeymoon phase ending as soon as you lose the desired amount of weight and face the challenge of keeping it off once you return to "normal" life (life not on a "diet"). Being aware of the possibility, or rather the probability, of facing such an emotional shift can prepare you to deal with it.

Another notorious bump in the diet road comes when you feel you are following the nutritional and activity guidelines—basically doing everything right—but you are not losing weight. This is the bump of the weight plateau. Unfortunately, plateaus are more the rule than the exception in all weight-loss attempts. In other words, it is not a matter of *if*, but *when*. Experiencing a plateau can cause you to lose willpower and motivation. You may devise a powerful rationale for stopping the weight-loss program and then relapse into old, comfortable behaviors. The keys to getting through a plateau are identifying its specific causes and adapting strategies for overcoming them. Let us discuss these challenges now and the strategies you can use to overcome them.

Weight Plateaus

There are many reasons you might initially lose weight and then stop. The following are the most common.

1. Fat has been replaced by muscle.

For most people, the bathroom scale provides the evidence of their weight loss. If the scale shows pounds dropping away, you feel successful and happy. If it does not, then you feel discouraged and frustrated, even panicked. While the scale can gauge your weight loss, it cannot gauge the change in your body composition. Exercise changes body composition. When you go from sedentary to active, your body responds by increasing the size of many of your muscles. You might look thinner, but the scale might show you are not losing weight. Why? Because a *pound of muscle takes up to seven times less space than a pound of fat!* So when the needle on the scale is not moving downward but your clothes are fitting more loosely, celebrate! You are probably losing fat and gaining muscle.

2. Fluid retention

If you are not getting enough fluid throughout the day, your body will often respond by retaining the fluid it has. As counterintuitive as it sounds, a well-hydrated body is less likely to retain fluids. So your first order of business when hitting a weight-loss plateau is to become conscious of your water intake. If it is low, increase it. If it is not, then consider some of the other causes of fluid retention: hot weather, sunburn, premenstrual bloating, and certain medications.

3. Adaptations to calorie deficit and calorie burning

As your body gets smaller, it adapts by needing fewer calories. Remember earlier in the program when you figured your current calorie needs (by multiplying your weight by 12)? As your weight changes, you will periodically need to recalculate your calorie needs. If you weigh 150 at first calculation and then lose 20 pounds, when you recalculate for a weight of 130, you will discover that your body requires 200 fewer calories per day. In other words, what it once took for you to *lose* weight may now be what it takes to *maintain* weight.

Another adaptation that occurs relates to your activity levels. If you do the same type of exercise every day, for the same amount of time or the same intensity, your body becomes efficient at burning calories within this routine. By including various types of exercises and activities in your exercise program or by increasing the duration or intensity of your current one, your body will be forced to use different muscles or the same muscles in different ways, thereby burning more calories.

4. Lack of Observation

Remember my favorite word? *Conscious!* If you are not committed to staying alert to changes in your body and emotions, or if you deny or ignore the "facts," then you may be misinterpreting what is happening in your weight-loss effort. You may think you are doing everything right, but you actually may be eating more or exercising less than you realize. Don't be hard on yourself if you find this to be true. Most of us experience lapses in willpower or moments when we make excuses or rationalize ourselves into less than great choices. That is why keeping records of what you eat, measuring portions, and recording activity in a log are so important. They help keep you focused and alert to the choices you are making.

Risk Factors Leading to Plateaus

Several factors can lead to weight-loss plateaus.

1. Negative Emotional States

Losing your motivation, your "great attitude," during a lifestyle change of any kind is not only a probability, it is, in all truth, a certainty. These periods of negativity or lapses in motivation can be both the *cause* and the *result* of weight plateaus. When you are down emotionally, you may decide to retreat to former unhealthy habits and the comfort provided by your old, favorite (and usually high-fat) food. The result is you will stop losing weight. On the other hand, if you stop losing weight because you are gaining muscle but do not realize that is the cause, you could become discouraged and give up. Either way the answer is to remain conscious, to monitor your emotional state as often as you monitor your weight loss.

2. Decreased Motivational Level

Losing your motivation may have nothing to do with a negative emotional state. It simply might be the result of reaching a preconceived goal. For example, your motivation for losing weight might have been to be able to wear your favorite bathing suit again. When October rolls around, what is going to keep you going in your new, healthier lifestyle? Or, say you were losing weight to please someone else and that person suddenly moves out of your life. Will your motivation vanish, too? It is important at the beginning of a weight-loss program to know what is motivating you. But when it comes to weight-management, it is just as important to continually find new, fresh motivations. Simply feeling healthier and more comfortable with your body can itself be a powerful motivation, but even the best of intentions need to be reinvigorated every now and again.

3. Inadequate social support

In Chapter 5 you examined how the relationships in your life might either help or hinder your efforts to improve your heath and lose weight. As those relationships or support systems shift and change, so can your weight-loss motivation and results. For example, perhaps you and your spouse started this program together, but your spouse has abandoned the effort. How will that affect your own effort? Or, maybe the friend with whom you shared an evening walk has moved out of the neighborhood. Will you continue to walk each night alone or with someone new? Change is inevitable, so it is important to have back-up plans for your original support strategies.

4. Lack of flexibility

Now that you know how to follow meal plans, count servings, and record your exercise, you might presume that the key to success is following the program perfectly. On the contrary, perfectionism often makes for rigidity rather than success. You might wish that the universe would surround you for the next several months with a magic bubble as a protection from upsetting events so that you can focus on your weight loss. In the real world that is just not going to happen. So, begin to anticipate how you will react when upsetting or disruptive events or emotions arise. Allow yourself the room to make mistakes and to recover from them. Instead of resisting change, be creative and learn to adapt to the new circumstances.

More Strategies for Overcoming Weight Plateaus

1. Be patient.

The reality is that plateaus can last for weeks or months. If you accept weight-loss plateaus as a part of the weight-loss process, you will reduce your feelings of failure. Eventually a plateau will break and weight loss will resume. In the meantime, measure your success by your lifestyle changes, not by the number on your scale.

2. Boost your metabolism.

The sure-fire way to boost your metabolism is to boost your strength training. Add an extra set, or challenge yourself to increase the amount of weight you are lifting if you can do so safely. Strong muscles are the foundation of your calorie-burning potential.

The worst thing you can do when you experience a plateau is to cut back on your food intake. Eating fewer calories may sound like a common sense and even an easy fix, but in the long run doing so will only make matters worse. When you reduce your food intake, your body goes into conservation mode, lowering its metabolism to conserve the calories it does obtain. Instead of cutting back, eat plenty of food that is high in nutrition and low in calories, such as fruits, vegetables, and whole grains. Also, stay in the habit of having small, frequent meals to keep your digestive engine humming.

3. Shake up your exercise program.

As mentioned earlier, your body may have adapted to an exercise routine, burning fewer calories than it did initially. By changing your routine, you can wake up your muscles to a new calorie-burning level. Try different aerobic exercises, experiment with different walking routes by choosing a hilly route instead of a flat one, add an interval or two to your weight training, take an extra lap around the track. With the new indoor fitness centers that seem to be springing up everywhere, you can swim in the winter and cross-country ski in the summer, so there is no shortage of new activities to try. A lifestyle that is adventurous, full of variety, and always pleasurable is the key to keeping your activity level up and improving your calorie-burning potential.

4. Revisit your food intake.

If you have stopped measuring your food, go back to it for a few days to see if your "eyeballed" portions are the same as the measured portions. A few extra calories here and there will add up to pounds over time.

If you stopped keeping a food diary, start again. This tool is tried and true for getting you to check up on your eating habits. Be sure to monitor your intake of refined carbohydrates, as this is one area that often gets out of hand. You do not have to eliminate them, but keep in mind that you should be eating nutritiously most of the time and enjoying refined carbohydrates only as an occasional treat.

5. Have a good talk with yourself.

While there are many things in life that are out of our control, we can regain control of our emotions and our thinking processes. When things go wrong or you are not losing weight, it is time for a good talk between your basic and conscious selves. It is the emotional, basic self who becomes discouraged by weight plateaus. As your conscious self gains understanding of the reasons for a weight plateau, you can help your emotional self to regain its optimism. Once you are into the program, take the time to look back over the previous few months and focus on what you have accomplished. Even small strides add up to a winning run! Use positive self-talk and affirmations to get yourself back on track when you falter, and when you are up and at it again, congratulate yourself. Praise is good for the soul—and for your weight-loss motivation.

6. Focus on long-term and internal motivators.

The best motivators for your long-term success are those that do not come from other people or rely on external conditions or factors. Two of the most lasting motivators are the improvement in your own physical health and the good feelings you have when you are taking care of yourself. Put the scale away for a while and focus on enjoying the pleasure of meeting daily goals such as exercise, which will itself release brain chemicals that can lighten your mood. While short-term goals are important, do not get so caught up in them that you lose sight of the long-range ones. A small setback in a short-term weight-loss goal does not have to affect your ultimate, long-term success in improving your lifestyle and your health.

7. Find the support you need.

As pointed out earlier, if the people you relied upon when you began the program are no longer there to support you, it is time to come up with a back-up plan. Do not try to "go it alone." We all need the non-judgmental support of others. This is a major reason why group weight-loss programs are valuable. Look for a friend to walk with, call old friends to talk to, join an exercise class. There are many ways to get the support you need even when those you are closest to are not helping you with your program. And, while social support is crucial, remember that your most important relationship is with yourself.

8. Develop resiliency and adaptability.

Although I have already talked about flexibility in an earlier section, it is worth repeating; because of all the strategies mentioned, it is the most useful. The bottom line is that it is essential to be flexible when life does not go according to your plans—which it never seems to do for very long. This is why you were encouraged from Day 1 of the Meal Plans to make substitutions when you did not like or could not find a recommended food item. Being adaptable gives you power. It means you do not get so invested in the "negative" event that you cannot find a positive outcome. What are you going to do when you discover that you left your carefully prepared lunch on the counter at home? Or when your car is in the shop and you have no way of getting to the gym? If you are able to go with the flow, think creatively, and bounce back from the curve balls life throws, you will have acquired one of life's most valuable skills—adaptability. You know the old saying, "Hope for the best, prepare for the worst." Believe it! While it is wise to plan ahead and have back-up plans, if you find yourself in a situation where you don't, then your main tools will be to adapt, improvise, think creatively, and keep a positive spirit.

Intentional Plateaus

In the course of a weight-loss program, situations often come up that make continued weight loss difficult. You might have to go on an unexpected business trip or spend your days in the hospital with a sick relative. So your food choices will be limited. Perhaps you injured your knee and cannot continue your activity schedule. Or maybe you won a two-week cruise and you know you will not be able to totally resist the temptation of those lavish buffets. In these types of situations, you will need to shift your expectations. During certain times in your life you will have priorities other than losing weight. That is fine! But what you should not lose sight of is that while circumstances can get you off track for a while, when you are ready to get back on track you will find doing so much easier if you have not *gained* weight. So, when these times arise, as they occasionally will, rather than saying, "I'm off the diet and I'm not going to think about my weight," say instead, "It's time to take an intentional plateau break."

An *intentional plateau* is a slowing down or stopping of weight loss that you can plan for or that you are aware you are in the midst of. Your exercise routine, your food choices, your intentions and motivation— whatever it is that is affected at that time—are going to change tempo- rarily because of circumstances that may be beyond your control. At these times, cut yourself some slack, but also cut a deal with yourself! What's the deal? You may stop losing weight, but you will *not* start gaining it. In a sense, an intentional plateau is practicing for your later weight-mainte- nance lifestyle.

During an intentional plateau, your object is to maintain your weight. You will need to remain conscious of your food choices and portion sizes, and you will endeavor to be as active as you can. But because intentional plateaus often arise because of a crisis or other trying time in life, focus on your self-care first. By eating healthy meals and staying active, you will be nurturing your body so it can better deal with what may be a stressful situation *and* you will be maintaining your weight.

Weight Maintenance

When most people reach their intended goal weight, their common thought is, "I am now off this diet and can eat as I please." The problem with this way of thinking is that it causes 75 percent of dieters to regain the weight they lost within one year, and 95 percent within three years. The California Wine Country Diet does not end once you have reached your weight goal. The challenge at the weight-maintenance stage is to stay committed to your new lifestyle by not returning to the undesirable eating and activity patterns that contributed to your weight-control prob- lem in the first place. Weight maintenance means adopting a healthy lifestyle that *you* can live with, so the process and strategies will vary. What allows you to maintain your weight will be unique to you, just as your weight loss program was not exactly the same as it was for others. For example, you may have found that recognizing feeling full as a signal to stop eating is an important weight loss tool; whereas someone else may need to focus on slowing their rate of eating. You need to be creative and persistent in finding what works for you for the long haul.

There are four key steps for weight maintenance:

1. Set your weight-maintenance goal.
If you have reached your goal weight, you are probably seeing, if you weigh yourself regularly, that your weight continues to fluctuate by a few pounds. It pays to be mindful of that fluctuation. People who have successfully maintained their weight do not let their weight fluctuate more than five pounds in either direction. If your weight goal is 150, do not let your weight go lower than 145 or higher than 155.

2. Balance calories in and out.
With weight loss, you adapted to an eating and exercise pattern that created a calorie deficit. With weight maintenance, your goal is to create an eating and exercise pattern where the calories you consume equals the calories you burn. Your calorie intake will probably be lower than it was before losing weight because your now-smaller body needs fewer calories to maintain its weight. Multiply your current goal weight by 12. This will give you the number of calories you need to consume each day for weight maintenance.

3. Define your lifestyle behaviors for weight maintenance.
As mentioned before, what works for you is as individual as you are. Also what works for you to maintain your weight now may not work for you at a later time. Periodically reevaluating which lifestyle patterns give you the most support is essential to successful weight maintenance.

The National Weight Control Registry is an organization that tracks behaviors of thousands of people who have lost a significant amount of weight and kept it off. To enroll in NWCR you must have lost at least 30 pounds and kept it off for a year. The average weight loss of participants is actually 66 pounds, and most have kept it off for more than five and a half years. In a nutshell, the most important lifestyle patterns for weight maintenance adopted by this group have more to do with exercise than nutrition. However, most people (89 percent) use a combination of the two. The following list contains behaviors that successful NWCR maintainers have adopted in terms of nutrition and physical activity:

Nutrition:
Continued with low-fat, healthy carbohydrate eating.
Controlled their calorie intake.
Frequently monitored their portion sizes and hunger.
Ate small, frequent meals (5-6x/day).
Ate most meals at home.
Learned to eat in a way that can be maintained for life.
Watched what they ate 90 percent of the time.

Physical activity:
Exercised up to 60 minutes/day; 400 calories/day; 2,000 calories/week.
Exercised at moderate to high intensity. (Walking was the most popular mode of exercise.)
Made fitness fun, something they enjoy.
Made exercise a priority, not an option.

Keep this list as a guide to what can help you maintain your weight loss, recognizing what will work for you and you alone.

4. Have a relapse plan.
It is important to have a plan if your weight falls outside of the predetermined range or your caloric intake goes above what you need for maintenance. Otherwise, it can be easy to rationalize setting new limits and making weight gain a lot easier. Think of distinct actions that you know made the most impact on your ability to lose weight. It is these

same actions that will help you if you find yourself headed toward relapse. For example, keeping a food diary or reinforcing your support system may get you back on track.

The first three days of the California Wine Country Diet, which are called "Simple Start," were designed to help take off the two or three pounds that have a way of creeping back on during maintenance, especially around the holidays. Most of the meals during these three Simple Start days have ingredients you may already have at home, so they will not take a lot of planning or shopping. Going back on the weight-loss program for three days may be the only adjustment that you will need.

Knowing what actions to take in advance and using them if you go outside your weight range or determined calorie level will make it that much easier to return to your weight-maintenance goals. Plan some strategies now, so you will be prepared when you need to use them:

If I reach my weight range limits, my action steps will be:

1.

2.

3.

4.

Putting the steps into action

Now is the time to put these four steps together to summarize your weight maintenance plan.

My Weight Maintenance Plan

A. My weight-maintenance goal is _____ pounds with a fluctuation of _____ pounds.

B. The number of calories I need to maintain this weight is
   _____ per day.

C. The lifestyle behaviors that will most help me to maintain
   my weight include:

   1.

   2.

   3.

D. If my weight falls outside of my predetermined weight range,
   or my calories go above the limit I set in B above, I will do
   the following:

   1.

   2.

   3.

Final Considerations

While doing the research for my book *Choosing to Be Well,* I inter-
viewed people who had overcome poor health habits and made significant changes in their health status. I found that the common turning
point in each of their stories—as to why they had begun to take care of
themselves—was that they had finally accepted something about them-

selves or their life situation about which they had previously been in denial. One woman, for example, did not lose weight until she accepted that she was angry at her husband. Another person did not accept that his high-fat diet and 150-pound weight gain were serious threats to his health until he was faced with a diagnosis of diabetes. Once he accepted the reality of his situation he was finally able to embark on a healthful exercise and weight loss program.

Those of us in America are going through a similar process in regards to accepting the devastation to the health of this country's citizens caused by modern lifestyles. Acceptance does not mean that we approve of this situation but rather that we are finally looking at it with clear eyes. Every day our newspapers are filled with stories about the epidemic of obesity in both adults and children. We are finally starting to address this issue in our homes, our towns, and on the national level.

It is essential that we face the negative impact to our health caused by the following factors: a significant decrease in normal daily physical activity; the production of cheap, refined processed foods; the infrequency with which families eat at home together; and the stressful pace of modern life. We have lives in which there is no time for a leisurely meal with our families as we rush from our frantic workplace to our frantic after-work lives. We are so overwhelmed by the multitude of information and variety in our world that we retreat to the comfort of sameness in our food selections and our life patterns.

The California Wine Country Diet is a program that addresses all the above factors of modern life in a proactive way through the Wheel of Weight-Management. While it may have been simply the wish to lose weight that brought you to this point, by now you have seen just how integral the process of selecting, preparing, and eating food is to your relationship with yourself and others. As you begin to look ahead to the Forever After of your life, it is essential that you accept the need for continual attention to physical activity, the amount and nutritional content of the food you eat, and strategies for relaxing from life's stresses. Going along with the "natural flow" of modern life will lead you naturally to the diseases of modern life.

There is one other factor that should help to keep you motivated.

The miracles of modern medicine are such that you will probably live far longer than your ancestors did. What your life will be like and how healthy you will be in your later years will largely be determined by how you take care of yourself in the coming years. None of us can any longer afford to remain unconscious to the choices we make in our eating habits, activity levels, and overall lifestyles.

In the course of The California Wine Country Diet program, you have come to look at how your own emotional and lifestyle patterns have contributed to weight gain and made weight maintenance difficult in the past. You now have the tools to support yourself in all aspects of your life as you go forward from this point. While most of us cannot, and probably do not want to give up our modern conveniences, we certainly can learn valuable lessons from the simpler lives of past generations and from traditional cultures about how to take better care of ourselves.

By eating locally grown, seasonal, and preferably organic food, we not only improve our health but support our local farmers while helping to keep the environment cleaner. By preparing home-cooked dinners, we bring our families together and teach our children by example to lovingly take care of their own bodies. By consciously indulging in the bounty of food and wine, we have a chance to find some relief from the stress of daily life and to enhance the pleasures in our lives. By being a bit adventurous and increasing the variety in our lives, we add sparkle to every day. Let us work together to take care of ourselves, our children, and our planet. We are our own caretakers. My wish for you is that you become the best one that you can be.

And so we end where we began, with the Wheel of Weight-Management. Let it continue rolling through your life.

Nutrition
I am giving myself the foods I need to nourish my body.

Activity
I am enjoying an active life.

Practicality
I am simplifying my life through practicality.

Pleasure
I am slowing down and taking time to enjoy my life.

Relationships
My relationship with myself enhances my relationships with others.

Variety
My life continues to unfold in new and exciting ways as
I embrace variety.

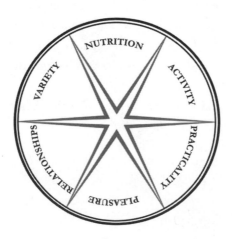

Acknowledgments

It was a fortunate day when I met Stephen Blake Mettee, publisher of Quill Driver Books/Word Dancer Press, at the Mendocino Coast Writers Conference in the summer of 2004. His clear understanding of the vision of this book and his consistent support for it has been an author's dream.

I am very grateful to John Ash for his willingness to write the Foreword. His leadership in developing California cuisine and the ethical food movement has been an inspiration to me. His perspective sheds light on how it is possible to attain a healthy weight while still nourishing ourselves in both body and soul.

The contributions of Sharon Stewart, M.S., R.D., have been invaluable to *The California Wine Country Diet.* Her knowledge and expertise in the fields of nutrition and physical activity have allowed me the freedom to focus on the areas of weight management that I know best. Sharon's hard work, flexibility, and enthusiasm for this project have been essential to its completion.

Getting feedback is a mixed blessing for a writer. You want people to love what you've written and yet you know you need the objective eyes of someone who is not afraid to give you their honest opinion. Joan Parisi Wilcox, a highly skilled writer and editor, has once again provided me with invaluable feedback and kept the book's focus where it should be—on its audience. I want to thank Jeff Brinkman, a winemaker who also has a degree in molecular and cellular biology, for his review of the chapter on wine. Finally, I want to express my appreciation to internist Sarah Ferguson, M.D., for her review of the medical and nutritional aspects of wine and other pleasure foods.

It was my husband, Robert Faulk, who originally came up with the idea of a diet based on California wine country cuisine. He has joined me in the delicious research for this book—the visiting of restaurants, wineries, and festivals throughout the wine country. He has shared with me the challenges and excitement of preparing the restaurant recipes at home. During each fabulous California Wine Country Diet dinner, we looked at each other in rapture and exclaimed that we had never eaten so well.

Another bonus of writing this book has been getting to spend more time with my childhood best friend, Ellen Holmes. Little did either of us imagine when we rode our bicycles back and forth to each other's houses sampling our favorite foods, that one day we would be working on recipes for a book together. To my good fortune, all the years when I was focusing on the problems of weight management, Ellen was perfecting her skills and knowledge about food and wine. Her testing of the recipes and advice on preparation has been invaluable. I also want to thank Jacqueline Granados and Geri Gugel for their recipe-testing, recipe ideas, and encouragement.

The gathering of restaurant recipes for the book has provided me with a glimpse into the world of chefs and restaurant managers. I am greatly appreciative of each and every one of them for taking the time in the midst their extremely busy lives to contribute recipes to *The California Wine Country Diet*. (Enjoy the experience of preparing these recipes at home and the delight of visiting their restaurants when you are in the area.)

My understanding of the emotional and social factors that impact weight management has come largely from the clients I have worked with over the past twenty-five years—I am grateful to all who have shared their struggles and successes with me.

I look forward to hearing about your adventures as you enjoy food, wine, and life while losing weight and then maintaining a healthy weight on the California Wine Country Diet.

Chapter Notes

Chapter 1 Nutrition:
Making Healthy Choices for Life

1. Thompson, Tommy G., Secretary of Health and Human Services, Press Release, January 12, 2005.
2. *Dietary Guidelines for Americans 2005*; Executive Summary, p. vi.
3. Ibid., p. vii.
4. *The Journal of the American Medical Association*, Vol. 292, No.12, September 22/ 29, 2004.
5. Department of Nutrition, Harvard School of Public Health, The Nutrition Source website, www.hsph.harvard.edu/nutritionsource, 2004.
6. *American Journal of Public Health*, 90 (5): 777-81, May 2000.

Chapter 2 Activity:
The Key to Permanent Weight Control

1. Mullen, Deborah, *Strength Training for Weight Loss Success*, www.simple fitnesssolutions.com, 2000.
2. "With understanding and improving health and objectives for improving health," *Healthy People 2010*. 2nd ed. 2 vols. Washington, DC: U.S. Government Printing Office, November 2000.
3. "A Focus on Obesity, Part 2," *The Permanente Journal*, Vol. 7, No. 3. Summer 2003.
4. Pavlou, KN; S Krey; and WP Steffee, "Exercise as an adjunct to weight loss and maintenance in moderately obese subjects," *American Journal of Clinical Nutrition*, 49: 1115S-1123S, 1989.
5. Brooks, George A. and Thomas D Fahey, *Exercise Physiology; Human Bioenergetics and Its Applications*, 1984.
6. Reprinted with the permission of the Canadian Society for Exercise Physiology, http://www.csep.ca
7. Booth, Michael L, "Assessment of Physical Activity: An International Perspective," *Research Quarterly for Exercise and Sport*, 71 (2): s114-120.
8. *Dietary Guidelines for Americans, 2005*, U.S. Department of Health and Human Services. U.S. Department of Agriculture, www.healthierus.gov/dietaryguidelines.
9. Ainsworth, G; W Haskell; et al., "Compendium of Physical Activities: Classification of energy costs of human physical activities," *Medicine Science in Sports and Exercise*, 23 (1):71-80, 1993.
10. Campbell, WW; MC Crim; VR Young; and WJ Evans, "Increased energy requirements and changes in body composition with resistance training in older adults," *American Journal of Clinical Nutrition* 60: 167-175, 1994.
11. Nelson, ME; WJ Evans; et al., "Effects of high intensity strength training on multiple risk factors for osteoporotic fractures. A randomized controlled trial," *Journal of the American Medical Association* 272: 1909-14, 1994.
12. Tremblay, A; J Simoneau; and C Bouchard, "Impact of exercise intensity on body fatness and skeletal muscle metabolism," *Metabolism.* 43:814-818, 1994.

Chapter 3 Practicality:
Finding What Works in Your Real Life

1. Finkelstein, Eric, *Obesity Research,* January 2004
2. Thomas, Paul R, Editor, *Weighing the Options*

Chapter 4 Pleasure:
The Sensual Side of Life

1. As reported on www.salary.com.
2. Urdang, Laurence, Editor in Chief, *The Random House College Dictionary*, 1972, p. 370.
3. Bozarth, Michael A, "Pleasure Systems in the Brain" in *Pleasure: the Politics and the Reality*, pp5-14.
4. Phillips, Helen, "The Pleasure Seekers," *New Scientist*, 11 October 2003.
5. Ibid.
6. Roth, Geneen, *Why Weight?: A Guide to Ending Compulsive Eating*, New York: Penquin Books USA, Inc., 1989, p.18.
7. Jenkins, Nancy Harmon, *The Mediterranean Diet Cookbook: a Delicious Alternative for Lifelong Health*, New York: Bantam Books, 1994, p. 489.

Chapter 5 Relationships:
How Family and Friends Can Support or Sabotage Us

1. Stuart, Richard B and Barbara Jacobson, *Weight, Sex and Marriage: A Delicate Balance*, pp 42–43.
2. Ibid, pp. 50–66.
3. American Academy of Pediatrics, "Prevention of Pediatric Overweight and Obesity," Volume 112, Number 2, August 2003, p. 427.

Chapter 6 Variety:
Our Need for Adventure and Change

1. *Seasonal Chef*, www.seasonalchef.com, "Nurturing Connections with Farmers: An Interview with Alice Waters," 1997.

Chapter 7:
Starting Your Activity Program

1. American College of Sports Medicine; American Dietetic Association; and Dietitians of Canada, "Joint Position Statement:Nutrition and Athletic Performance," *Medicine and Science in Sports and Exercise*, 2000.
2. Levine, James A.; Lanningham-Foster, Lorraine M.; McCrady, Shelly K.; Krizan, Alisa C.; Olson, Leslie R.; Kane, Paul H.; Jensen, Michael D.; and Clark, Matthew M. " Interindividual Variation in Posture Allocation: Possible Role in Human Obesity," *Science* 28: 584-586, January 2005.
3. American College of Sports Medicine, "Calculate Your Exercise Heart Rate Range," www.acsm.org.

4. American College of Sports Medicine, "Guidelines for Graded Exercise Testing and Exercise Prescription," Philadelphia: Lea & Febiger, 1986.
5. U.S. Department of Health and Human Services, U.S. Department of Agriculture, "Dietary Guidelines for Americans 2005," www.healthierus.govdietary guidelines.
6. Liebenson, Craig, "Balance Exercises," The Gym Ball Store, www.gymball.com.
7. Janda V., et al., "Sensory motor stimulation" in Liebenson, C. (ed), *Spinal Rehabilitation: A Manual of Active Care Procedures.* Williams and Wilkins, Baltimore, 1996.
8. Moore, M.A.; Hutton, R.S., "Electromyographic Investigation of Muscle Stretching Techniques," *Medicine and Science in Sports and Exercise,* 12:322-329, 1980.
9. Morrissey, M.C.; Harman, E.A.; Frykman, P.N.; and Han, K.H., "Early phase differential effects of slow and fast barbell squat training," *The American Journal of Sports Medicine* 26:221-230, 1998.
10. Lachance, Peter F.; and Hortobagyi, Tibor, "Influence of cadence on muscular performance during push-up and pull-up exercises," *The Journal of Strength and Conditioning Research*: 8:76-79, 1994.
11. Hay, J.G.; Andrews, J.G.; and Vaughan, C.L., "Effects of lifting rate on elbow torques exerted during arm curl exercises," *Medicine and Science in Sports and Exercise,* 15:63-71, 1993.
12. www.fitnessjournal.org.

Chapter 8:
Getting Ready to Start the Daily Meal Plans

1. National Institutes of Health; National Heart, Lung, and Blood Institute, *Evidence Report of Clinical Guidelines on the Identification, Evaluation, and Treatment of Overweight and Obesity in Adults,* NIH Publication No. 98-4083, September 1998.
2. Ibid.
3. Neiman, David C, *The Sports Medicine Fitness Course,* p. 187.
4. United States Department of Health and Human Services and United States Department of Agriculture, adapted from *Dietary Guidelines for Americans, 2005.*
5. Freedman, Marjorie; Janet King; and Eileen Kennedy, "Popular Diets: A Scientific Review," *Obesity Research*, Volume 9, Supplement 1, March 2001.

Chapter 11:
Wine and Other Pleasure Foods

1. "The Sweet Story of Chocolate" in *Light & Tasty*, February-March 2005, p. 65.
2. Rinzler, Carol Ann, *Nutrition for Dummies*, 3rd Edition, 358-359.
3. Netzer, Corrine T, *The Complete Book of Food Counts*, Sixth Edition. Calorie counts of favorite Pleasure Foods were selected from the lists in this book.
4. Phillips, Rod, *A Short History of Wine.*
5. Hardesty, Kathy Marcks, "Alcohol and Health," in *Vine Times*, January 2004, p. 33.
6. Interview with Dr. Eric Rimm, "Alcohol and Health: Medical Evidence" in *Alcohol & Health Issues*, 9-5-04.

7. Kahn, HS et al., "Stable Behaviors Associated with Adults' 10-year Change in Body Mass Index and Likelihood of Gain at the Waist, *American Journal of Public Health*, 1997; 87 (5): 747-754.

8. Rayyis, Jamal A. *Food & Wine Magazine's Wine Guide 2005*, p. 14-23.

9. Immer, Andrea, *Great Wine Made Simple*.

10. Ash, John, *From the Earth to the Table*, 381-395.

11. Sims, Fiona, *Guide to Wine*, 46-53.

12. Drake, Andrea, "Pairing Food with Wine," article on www.westcoastwine.net.

13. Berger, Eric, "Sugary Drinks Sour Health of U.S. Women" in the *Houston Chronicle*, August 25, 2004.

14. Severson, Kim, "Fine Dining, Hold the Alcohol," *The New York Times*, as reported in *The Press Democrat*, March 9, 2005.

15. As reported by Jeff Brinkman, winemaker and former skin cancer researcher.

16. Rinzler, Carol Ann, *Nutrition for Dummies*, 3rd Edition, p. 359.

Suggested Reading and Resources

Reading

American Heart Association. *Fitting in Fitness: Hundreds of Simple Ways to Put More Physical Activity into Your Life.* New York: Random House, 1997.

Ash, John, with Amy Mintzer. *John Ash Cooking One on One: Private Lessons in Simple, Contemporary Food from a Master Teacher.* New York: Clarkson Potter, 2004.

Ash, John, with Sid Goldstein. *From the Earth to the Table.* New York: Penguin Group, 1995.

Binns, Brigit L. *Williams-Sonoma Hors D'Oeuvre.* New York: Simon & Schuster, 2001.

Bortz, M.D., Walter M., Sharon Bortz, R.D., and Patricia Mathis, R.N., *Diabetes Weight Loss System.* Washington, D.C.: Diabetes Research & Wellness Foundation, 1999.

Bozarth, Michael A. Pleasure Systems in the Brain. In D.M. Warburton (ed.) *Pleasure: The Politics and the Reality.* New York: John Wiley & Sons, 1994.

Brooks, George A. and Thomas D. Fahey. *Exercise Physiology: Human Bioenergetics and Its Applications.* New York: John Wiley & Sons, 1984.

Colvin, Robert H., Ph.D. and Susan C. Olson, Ph.D. *Keeping It Off: Winning at Weight Loss.* Arkansas City, KS: Gilliland, 1989.

Dolan, Paul, with Thom Elkjer. *True to Our Roots: Fermenting a Business Revolution.* Princeton: Bloomberg Press, 2003.

Doppenberg, Jean Saylor. *Insiders' Guide® to California's Wine Country: Including Napa, Sonoma, Mendocino, and Lake Counties.* Guilford, CT: The Globe Pequot Press, 2003.

Guiliano, Mireille. *French Women Don't Get Fat.* New York: Alfred A. Knopf, 2005.

Halm, Meesha, Maura Sell, and Troy Segal. *Zagat Survey® 2004 San Francisco Bay Area Restaurants.* New York: Zagat Survey, LLC, 2004.

Herbst, Sharon Tyler. *Food Lover's Companion: Comprehensive Definitions of Nearly 6000 Food, Drink, and Culinary Terms.* Hauppauge, N.Y.: Barron's Educational Series, Inc., 2001.

Hutchinson, Ed.D., Marcia Germaine. *Transforming Body Image: Learning to Love the Body You Have.* Freedom, CA: The Crossing Press, 1985.

Immer, Andrea. *Everyday Dining with Wine.* New York: Broadway Books, 2004.

————. *Great Wine Made Simple: Straight Talk from a Master Sommelier.* New York: Broadway Books, 2000.

Jenkins, Nancy Harmon. *The Mediterranean Diet Cookbook: A Delicious Alternative for Lifelong Health.* New York: Bantam Books, 1994.

Jordan, Michele Anna. *California Home Cooking: American Cooking In the California Style.* Boston, MA: The Harvard Common Press, 1997.

Knickerbocker, Peggy. *Olive Oil: From Tree to Table.* San Francisco: Chronicle Books, 1997.

Kochilas, Diane. *Meze.* New York: Harper Collins, 2003.

Logan, Ph.D., Haven. *Choosing to Be Well: A Conscious Approach to a Healthier Lifestyle.* Makawao, HI: Inner Ocean, 2002.

Louden, Jennifer. *The Woman's Comfort Book: A Self-Nurturing Guide for Restoring Balance in Your Life.* San Francisco: Harper San Francisco, 1992.

Martin, Don W. and Betty Woo Martin. *The Best of the Wine Country: An Opinionated and Remarkably Useful Guide to California's Vinelands.* Las Vegas, NV: Discover Guides, 2002.

Netzer, Corinne T. *The Complete Book of Food Counts, Sixth Edition.* New York: Random House, 2003.

Neiman, David C., D.H.Sc. *The Sports Medicine Fitness Course.* Palo Alto, CA: Bull Publishing Company, 1986.

Pennington, Ph.D., Jean A.T., revised by. *Bowes and Church's Food Values of Portions Commonly Used, 15th Edition.* New York: Harper Collins Publishers, 1989.

Pert, Ph.D., Candace B. *Molecules of Emotion: Why You Feel the Way You Feel.* New York: Simon & Schuster, 1997.

Petusevsky, Steve and Whole Foods Market Team Members. *The Whole Foods Market® Cookbook: A Guide to Natural Foods with 350 Recipes.* New York: Clarkson Potter Publishers, 2002.

Rayyis, Jamal A. *Food & Wine Magazine's Wine Guide 2005.* New York: American Express Publishing Corporation, 2004.

Rinzler, Carol Ann. *Nutrition for Dummies, 3rd Edition.* Hoboken, N.J.: Wiley Publishing, Inc., 2004.

Roth, Geneen. *When Food Is Love: Exploring the Relationship Between Eating and Intimacy.* New York: Penguin Group, 1991.

————. *Why Weight?: A Guide to Ending Compulsive Eating.* New York: Penguin Books USA Inc., 1989.

Simon, Joanna. *Discovering Wine: A Refreshingly Unfussy Beginner's Guide to Finding, Tasting, Judging, Storing, Serving, Cellaring, and Most of All, Discovering Wine.* New York: Simon & Schuster, 2003.

Simopoulos, M.D., Artemis P. and Jo Robinson. *The Omega Diet: The Lifesaving Nutritional Program Based on the Diet of the Island of Crete.* New York: Harper Collins Publishers, 1999.

Sims, Fiona. *Guide to Wine: An Introduction for Beginners.* East Sussex, United Kingdom: The Bridgewater Book Company, Ltd., 2001.

Stuart, Richard B. and Barbara Jacobson. *Weight, Sex and Marriage: A Delicate Balance.* New York: Simon & Schuster, Inc., 1989.

Thomas, Paul R., editor. *Weighing the Options: Criteria for Evaluating Weight-Management Programs.* Washington, D.C.: National Academy Press, 1995.

Weil, M.D., Andrew and Rosie Daley. *The Healthy Kitchen: Recipes for a Better Body, Life, and Spirit.* New York: Alfred A. Knopf, 2003.

Weir, Joanne. *Joanne Weir's More Cooking in the Wine Country.* New York: Simon & Schuster, 2001.

Whitney, Eleanor Noss, Corinne Balog Cataldo, Sharon Rady Rolfes. *Understanding Normal and Clinical Nutrition, Fifth Edition.* Belmont, CA: West/Wadsworth, 1998.

Web Sites

www.acsm.org (American College of Sports Medicine)

www.almanac.com (The Old Farmer's Almanac)

www.californiacoastalwines.com

www.californiawinecountrydiet.com
(official website for this book where you can download the
Daily Meal Plan form)

www.chefscollaborative.org

www.chefjohnash.com

www.cookinglight.com

www.chowhound.com

www.fitnessjournal.org (online exercise log)

www.foodandwine.com

www.foodreference.com

www.foodtv.com (lots of recipes and listings for cooking shows)

www.geneenroth.com

www.healthierus.gov/dietaryguidelines
(USDA Dietary Guidelines 2005 and new food pyramids)

www.iacp.com (International Association of Culinary Professionals)

www.inwinecountry.com (weekly television show)

www.localharvest.org (nationwide directory of small farms,
farmers' markets, and other local food sources)

www.madeincalifornia.net

www.nbc11.com (look for weekly "In Wine Country" show)

www.oldwayspt.org (Oldways Preservation & Exchange Trust)

www.seasonalchef.com

www.seedsavers.org (Seed Savers Exchange)

www.simplefitnesssolutions.com

www.slowfoodusa.org

www.usawines.com

www.vinography.com

www.wine.com

www.winecountry.com

www.wineinstitute.org (California Wine Institute)

Index

About the Author

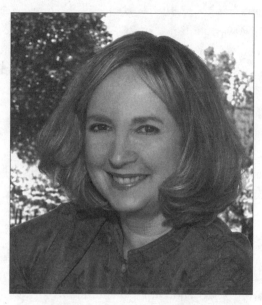

Haven Logan, Ph.D.

With *The California Wine Country Diet,* author Haven Logan, Ph.D. says that she has come full circle back to the joys of food she experienced as a child. She first learned to love food's many aspects through her father who was a gourmet chef and vice president of General Foods in charge of research and development. She relates that she looked forward to the nightly adventure of trying new delicacies, such as birds nest soup and dehydrated meats being tested for space flights, proudly proclaiming that "there was no food I wouldn't try."

Dr. Logan's educational background includes a B.A. in sociology from Barnard College at Columbia University, a master's degree in education from Bank Street College of Education, a master's degree in social work from the University of Southern California, and a Ph.D. in psychology from International College. As a psychotherapist and program director, she has specialized in the treatment of eating disorders and weight management for more than twenty years. She has spoken about these subjects to hundreds of groups, as well as to radio and television audiences.

Dr. Logan's book *Choosing to Be Well: A Conscious Approach to a Healthier Lifestyle* was published in 2002. This book explores the question of why people don't do the things they know they should for their health. *The California Wine Country Diet* makes choosing wellness a pleasure.

Sharon Stewart, M.S., R.D.

Sharon Stewart, M.S., R.D., is the consultant for the nutritional and exercise content of *The California Wine Country Diet*. A registered dietitian, Ms. Stewart received a master's degree in nutrition and applied physiology from Columbia University. She is a former research dietitian at the Stanford Center for Research in Disease Prevention and at Tufts University in Boston. She is the coauthor of *Diabetes Weight Loss System* (as Sharon Bortz) and author of numerous articles and programs on nutrition, fitness, and weight loss. She has a private practice in Ukiah, California.